Risky Medicine

Risky Medicine

Our Quest to Cure
Fear and Uncertainty

Robert Aronowitz

The University of Chicago Press
Chicago and London

Robert Aronowitz is professor and chair of the history and sociology of science at the University of Pennsylvania; he earned his medical degree from Yale University. His books include *Making Sense of Illness: Science, Society, and Disease* and *Unnatural History: Breast Cancer and American Society*. He lives in Merion Station, Pennsylvania.

The University of Chicago Press, Chicago 60637
The University of Chicago Press, Ltd., London
© 2015 by The University of Chicago
All rights reserved. Published 2015.

Printed in the United States of America

24 23 22 21 20 19 18 17 16 15   1 2 3 4 5

ISBN-13: 978-0-226-04971-7   (cloth)
ISBN-13: 978-0-226-04985-4   (e-book)
DOI: 10.7208/chicago/9780226049854.001.0001

Library of Congress Cataloging-in-Publication Data
Aronowitz, Robert A. (Robert Alan), 1953– author.
  Risky medicine : our quest to cure fear and uncertainty / Robert Aronowitz.
    pages cm
  Includes bibliographical references and index.
  ISBN 978-0-226-04971-7 (cloth : alkaline paper) — ISBN 978-0-226-04985-4 (e-book)
1. Medicine, Preventive—United States—History—20th century. 2. Diseases—Risk factors—Social aspects—United States. 3. Medical care—United States—History—20th century. I. Title.
  R151.A76 2015
  610.28'9—dc23

                                                              2015012605

♾ This paper meets the requirements of ANSI/NISO Z39.48-1992 (Permanence of Paper).

Contents

I

1

Risky medicine: Our quest to cure fear and uncertainty

On the front page of the *New York Times* the day I was first drafting this introductory chapter was a story about how a National Cancer Institute working group had recommended that some carcinomas in situ and cancers of low metastatic potential be renamed without the word *cancer* in them.[1] Removing *cancer* would by fiat decrease the overdiagnosis of cancer but also might reduce fear and overtreatment.

The overdiagnosis and overtreatment of cancer is part of a larger cost and quality crisis in American medicine today. American health care is more intensive and costly, but our health is the same or worse, than countries which do less and spend less. The modest proposal to rename disease is an imaginative response to one driver of this crisis: the high numbers of Americans who are diagnosed with "early" stages of disease and risk states yet treated as full-blown disease, triggering fear as well as aggressive and costly treatments whose net benefits are often assumed rather than proven.

Unfortunately, our policy responses to what ails American medicine are usually not so imaginative, and have been focused almost exclusively on the organization and financing of health services. We need to reform the way we deliver and pay for care, but these are not the only problems and solutions. In this book I want to draw attention to a profound and consequential historical transformation in our illness experience and medical and public health practices that contributes to many of our health care woes. We have experienced the ascent of a *risk-dominated* experience of ill health, one characterized by fear, uncertainty, and lack of control, whereas in the past, pain, loss of function, and other symptoms were more central. Along with this, we have more and more public health practices, medical interventions, and consumer products that are largely *risk reducing* and *risk controlling* rather than treating symptoms or curing disease.

In the chapters that follow, I will explain how risk became central to the experience of health and medical interventions and flesh out some of the implications of this transformation. While the experience of illness and medical practices have been radically transformed in recent decades, our individual and collective responses have not kept up with these changes. Failure to appreciate these changes has led to wasted resources, hits to our health and peace of mind, and myopic solutions to our cost/quality crisis.

Current received wisdom is that the unaffordable yet underperforming U.S. health care system is due to a number of factors: new technology; greedy practitioners, drug companies, device manufacturers, and health systems; hyperspecialization; inadequate evaluation of medical practices and products; malpractice concerns; and fee-for-service reimbursement. But underlying and contributing to the creation and diffusion of new technologies and shaping demand for services and products, irrespective of work force, legal, or financial arrangements, are changes in how we have defined, labeled, researched, and responded to ill health and its putative causes.

There are three key aspects of this risk-centered medicine that I will sometimes refer to as *risky medicine* when I invoke these ideas together. One is the *market-driven expansion of risk interventions*, especially drugs and screening tests (chapter 9). Drugs that cure or ameliorate disease have limited markets. Any particular disease affects only a minority, usually a small minority, of the population. Disease may be self-limited, or worse, from the perspective of pharmaceutical companies' bottom-line, quickly cured by drugs. In contrast, an entire population can be at risk for even a rare disease and be convinced to take a disease-reducing drug for life. For example, cholesterol-lowering drugs aimed at reducing the risk of heart disease and stroke might be indicated for a large fraction of a population for their entire life span. Second is the *converged experience of risk and disease*. Developments on many levels, within and outside of medicine, have transformed the experience of many chronic diseases into one of intensive surveillance and anticipatory treatment and behavioral change (chapter 2). Third is the way we increasingly understand and accept that many medical and public health interventions are *efficacious because they reduce risk* and do social and psychological work (chapter 3).

At the outset, let me be clear that elements of *risky medicine* have always been part of the illness experience.[2] Medical interventions have long targeted the anticipated consequences of specific diseases. But changes in how we understand, name, classify, screen for, and treat disease have made the risk-centered experience of ill health dominant for a much larger proportion of Americans. This experience has been infused with probabilistic knowledge of potential bad outcomes and medical interventions that promise to modify them.

It is also self-evident that the same medical progress that has contributed to decreased mortality and morbidity has also contributed to the growth of new risks and risk interventions. No one wants to set back the clock to the era before insulin, even though as more type 1 diabetics escaped death from acute episodes of high blood sugar (as in diabetic ketoacidosis) they lived at greater risk of heart and kidney damage and a host of other problems. But recognizing and celebrating this trade-off is not a reason to eschew critical examination of every new medical risk and intervention that emerges within the penumbra of medical progress. In diabetes, for example, we have had a problematic promotion of "prediabetes" risk states and calls for preventative treatment.

In making disease, especially chronic disease, *risk-centered*, we have spawned interventions that do all kinds of work, such as providing reassurance, reducing fear, and signaling responsibility for health (chapter 3). Risk-reducing interventions—calls for behavioral change, screening, preventative drugs—are increasingly prevalent. Their efficacy is necessarily understood in a different way than practices that directly and immediately impact symptoms from, or signs of, disease. Their efficacy often involves some leap of faith, requiring trust in results of epidemiological or clinical research. Practitioners, patients, and consumers at the same time need some witnessed evidence of efficacy—reports of lowered cholesterol, improvements on bone densitometry, or images of healthy bowels. At a more psychological level, efficacy is often constituted by reduction in fear, banishing uncertainty, and reasserting some control over feelings of randomness. Risk-reducing interventions and risks themselves are often co-constructed and together constitute a coherent if largely invisible system of belief and practice.[3] This system, often loosely tethered to any specific knowledge production of medical evidence per se, often undergirds efficacy calculations.

This social and psychological work is a major reason why American medicine is so costly and yet not that effective when measured by objective impacts on morbidity and mortality. It creates incentives and provides a rationale for different stakeholders to make decisions divorced from objective impact on bodies and populations. This problem exists for highly visible and often controversial medicalized risk interventions such as drugs to reduce obesity or certain cancer screening tests, but also in less visible and controversial interventions aimed at preventing complications of existing chronic disease.

Many of the current ineffective or costly but marginally effective health practices are risk interventions that have not been adequately recognized, named, or understood. Unless we understand the scope of this change and the historically conditioned processes that undergird them, we will continue to engage in short-sighted after-the-fact policy debates about singular primary or secondary prevention practices, missing the bigger picture and "upstream" opportunities for policy change (chapter 9). The disease prevention landscape has been radically transformed over the past half-century, but our health policies and clinical practices have not been based on an adequate knowledge of this transformation. Health risks dominate medical practice, yet are poorly acknowledged. Demand for risk interventions has been heavily influenced by direct marketing to consumers, the sometimes exaggerated claims of self-interested parties, and problematic assumptions used in the extrapolation of aggregate data to individual decisions.

Understanding the history and reach of the transformed disease experience also provides a much-needed context for consumers, patients, and doctors making difficult health decisions under great uncertainty. A friend of mine was recently diagnosed with prostate cancer after one of twenty blind ultrasound-directed biopsies was positive. The biopsies were triggered by an elevated result on a screening blood test for the prostate specific antigen (PSA), which was added—

without any discussion—to his "routine" blood work during an annual visit to his primary care physician. Presented by his urologist with the choice of surgery, radiation, or active surveillance, my friend chose the last. A year after his diagnosis, my friend returned to the urologist for a follow-up visit. The urologist told him that although his PSA level had actually fallen in each of the two postbiopsy visits, he wanted, as part of an active surveillance protocol, to do another set of biopsies. My friend, puzzled and confused, politely said no. The urologist initially tried to change my friend's mind, but after a while gave up, saying it was in the end my friend's choice whether to actively monitor and potentially intervene in and cure his cancer or choose *palliation*.

The choice of the latter term struck my friend as especially odd. Why invoke palliation, which in the context of cancer typically means treating pain and other symptoms in the last phases of disease? My friend had simply calculated that the possible harms of more needles and what might follow outweighed the very small chance he might suffer health consequences from waiting a while before more probing. In one sense, there was a disagreement between my friend and his urologist over probabilities and outcomes, the values and utilities associated with a particular medical procedure. But in another more profound sense, my friend and his urologist were living on different sides of a historical transformation. My friend was resisting further involvement in a dense web of surveillance, risk assessment, and interventions that had been triggered by a routine blood test within a routine exam—none of which would have happened a half century ago. He was trying to take a few steps back to the time in which medical encounters were primarily the management of felt bodily experience and physical signs rather than highly probabilistic risk knowledge and states that increasingly are produced by medically directed surveillance and probing.

But to his urologist, my friend suffered from a *real* disease, "early" prostate cancer, and to abandon active surveillance was equivalent to giving up on the possibility of cure—thus his reference to *palliation*. This conflict is typically understood in a piecemeal way, as a set of individual medical problems that will be ameliorated by more and better evidence, or by system-wide reforms to decrease the biases and incentives that lead to costly, ineffective care. But we miss an opportunity to both better understand and respond when we ignore the underlying historical conditions that have transformed diseases and diagnoses, medical work, and patienthood. The chapters that follow explore the reasons for and the nature and consequences of these transformations.

In tracing these transformations, I aim to contribute to the history and sociology of medicine, in particular the study of disease and the disease experience, as well as to our thinking about policy choices. Part 1 of the book (this introductory chapter and the next two chapters) includes wide-angle essays on the converged experience of risk and disease and the efficacy of risk interventions. Part 2 (chapters 4–8) contains focused case studies of the history and sociology of particular risk research programs and interventions and risk experiences. Part 3 (chapters 9 and 10) draws some clinical and policy implications of the historical transformations that constitute *risky medicine*.

I explore in chapter 5, for example, the details and implications of the new HPV vaccines' co-construction as vaccines against cancer and as proprietary drugs that promise to reduce and control individual risk. This dual identity explains these vaccines' architecture, perceived efficacy, cost, and marketing. HPV infection has been constructed as a risk state or experience. The vaccines promise not only to prevent cervical cancer and other disease outcomes, but this state or experience of HPV risk. The HPV vaccines' differences from traditional vaccines may be difficult to appreciate because researchers, public health officials, drug manufacturers, and clinicians have blurred the border between risk and disease and have appropriated older rationales and the language of traditional clinical interventions and public health for new ends.

In chapter 6, I explore the history of the two vaccines against Lyme disease (LD) that were developed and tested in the 1990s. Despite pre-marketing evidence of their safety and efficacy, one was withdrawn prior to regulatory review and the other after only three years on the market. The history of these vaccines illuminates the challenges faced by many new risk-reducing products and practices and underscores the importance of their social and psychological, as distinct from biomedical or scientific, efficacy in their initial promise and later failure.

Then, in chapter 7, I explore the rapid growth and changing meaning of cancer survivorship, one of the most prominent examples of the converged experience of risk and disease. Long-term survivorhood is no longer a period of receding worry after cancer diagnosis and treatment. Knowledge of risks emanating from the natural history of cancer and previous cancer interventions has led to many new types of often intense surveillance and intervention. There have been some problematic consequences of this transformation. As many more people become cancer survivors due to expansion of the diagnosis and creation of new precancerous and at-risk conditions, people with rapidly growing and difficult-to-treat cancer have less societal visibility. They represent a much smaller fraction of the total number of people labeled as having cancer. Some interventions "work" not so much to improve a survivor's life chances as to restore control and certainty to the risk-dominated survival experience.

Overall, the book focuses on aspects of risk that are controversial and contribute to dilemmas in policy maker, physician, patient, and consumer decision making, and in which some gap exists between medical and consumer appeal and existing scientific evidence. But this focus on the downsides of risk-centered disease prevention and chronic disease management courts a very real danger—throwing out effective preventive or disease-modifying intervention, i.e., the baby, with problematic risk intervention bathwater. Despite this danger, I spend little time discussing the upsides of medical prevention and risk intervention. This is partly because I do not want to clutter the narrative with repeated observations that some primary and secondary prevention is effective, which is of course true, when calling attention to it serves only to provide rhetorical balance. But I also believe that the commonsense appeal of prevention, along with many vested interests and problematic values I explore in these chapters, has contributed to our inertia in grappling with and recognizing the implications of the changes I describe. Some of the concerns I raise are readily dismissed as the necessary, if unfortunate, cost of doing the business of effective disease prevention. I worry that the constant and automatic fealty to the self-evident benefits of disease prevention has rationalized many interventions we might better have jettisoned or prevented from diffusing prior to rigorous evaluation. So the chapters that follow often dispense with the conventional nod to the obvious positive impact of some disease prevention efforts, such as our mandated childhood vaccines and taking aspirin after heart attacks.

While effective disease prevention is obviously an important goal of medicine, a good deal of current risk intervention is wasteful and problematic. Many people bemoan the lack of high-quality evidence for the efficacy of many current medical interventions. But it is not always sufficiently appreciated that many risk interventions often diffuse through the population prior to, or independent of, evidence of efficacy because of the compelling and seemingly self-evident logic of identifying risk factors or early stages of disease and the persuasive power of witnessed evidence of risk reduction or elimination of a risk factor or the bit of the body containing early disease. Looked at this way, the absence of evidence is more of a permissive condition than a cause of the current disease prevention landscape's many costly but ineffective or marginally effective risk interventions.

At the same time, the adoption and diffusion of risk interventions without solid evidence of scientific efficacy is often much more consequential than other medical interventions. They are often mass interventions that spread through the population and resist challenge because they reduce fear and restore control, i.e., they have large social and psychological impacts and are difficult to objectively evaluate and change once they are in place (chapter 3). Moreover, there is perhaps a greater ethical burden on clinical and public health authorities to evaluate the efficacy of risk interventions, as they often involve individuals who are recruited and persuaded to participate and who prior to medical encounters may have had no symptoms or complaints. Given these considerations, there is more reason to have a "show me" vigilance and a high threshold for good scientific evidence of efficacy before allowing risk knowledge and interventions to gain traction. And given the cacophony of voices and interests in the medical marketplace, risk interventions are perhaps that part of modern medicine most in need of a respected centralized authority to evaluate them and suggest policy responses.

Complicating risk-related policy responses is that what makes sense for countries in one part of the world may not be the best course for other parts. In chapter 8, I explore some of the challenges that follow when disease prevention and intervention ideas and practices developed in rich countries with their particular social and scientific efficacies circulate to poor parts of the world (as well as a few examples of reverse circulation).

II

At first glance, the argument in *Risky Medicine* might seem a variant of a more familiar one about medicalization. However, it differs from accounts of the problematic growth of, say, attention deficit disorder or social anxiety disorder (aka shyness) by focusing on the transformation of *existing* disease categories and the expansion of *disease-focused* treatments as well as the intrusion of new medical diagnoses into the realm of the previously healthy. Historians, sociologists, cultural and medical critics, and journalists working within the medicalization paradigm have generally not recognized, understood, or explained the full implications of what I am calling the converged experience of risk and disease. This convergence is in part a medicalization story, but in large measure traces a story going in the opposite direction, how the experience of symptomatic illness has been transformed into one dominated by interventions aimed at warding off anticipated complications.

Secondly, insofar as *Risky Medicine* overlaps with some medicalization scholarship and popular accounts, it does so with the ambition of giving a sociohistorical explanation for a new logic and economy of risk, one that results in risk interventions for entire populations throughout their life span.[4] I have also observed that many of our current policy and clinical problems are the results not so much of bad actors (such as pharmaceutical companies and profit-maximizing practitioners and hospitals) but rather of the typical ways knowledge is produced and the values and interests that are the basis of everyday clinical practices and institutions. This makes the identification of both the problem and the solutions more complex, but that is not a reason to offer simpler analyses.

My argument is that many interventions that are understood as treating disease are essentially reducing the risk of some anticipated bad outcome. We treat diabetes largely to prevent end stage complications. Rheumatoid arthritis patients take disease-stabilizing drugs that promise a better disease trajectory more than immediate relief of symptoms. The families of Alzheimer's patients taking any of the currently offered medicines cannot expect their loved ones to actually get better—the promise is that people taking them will get worse more slowly than those who do not take them. We treat depression in some small measure to reduce the risk of suicide. Patients with minimally invasive cancers get systemic treatments because they are at risk for hidden disease elsewhere in their body. Chronic disease has been transformed but we respond, as patients, doctors, or public health agencies, with older assumptions and behaviors. These chapters tell the story of this transition to *risky medicine* and flesh out its implications.

III

While there have been steady improvements in objective health statistics (i.e., increased life expectancy) within industrialized countries throughout the twentieth century, I am suggesting that people often experience their own health as more fraught with uncertainty and difficult decisions, are more frequently diagnosed with risk factors and earlier stages of disease, and often experience more risk-related interventions. One reason for the ascendency of *risky medicine* is the explosion in knowledge about health risks, whose post–World War II seminal development, the Framingham Heart Study, I explore in chapter 4. In addition, the illness experience has become risky not only because mass risk interventions have medicalized the formerly healthy but also due to the increasing number of preventative interventions in chronic disease management (chapters 2 and 3).

The illness experience has also become more *risk-centered* in more material ways. In particular, changes in the built environment and other technological developments have led to more or at least different types of risks entering the body and being recognized and labeled as such. Perhaps the most important material way that risk became more central to the disease experience has been via consumer products and behaviors. These products and behaviors have coevolved with new medical risk categories, and are best understood as a package.

Much ill health in affluent societies has been associated with changing patterns of consumption.[5] It is well accepted that some commodities that get into the body (e.g., dietary fats) or are features of the built environment (e.g., unsafe neighborhoods) are risks for bad health outcomes. Less attention has been paid to how commodities are designed and marketed, and the processes by which particular products or patterns of consumption are framed as health problems or risks. Let me illustrate with an example from a recent case study.[6]

Schull carried out a largely ethnographic study of the relationship between the producers and consumers of video poker games.[7] She showed a complex interaction among the makers and users of game technologies that has led to subtle, often individualized manipulation of design elements that accommodates and creates complex and diverse consumer needs. As a result of these interactions, consumers spend more time and money on gaming and more consumers have, or are understood to have, a gaming addiction. The increased demand for, and use of, gaming technologies is thus understood as a health problem for a number of reasons. First, addiction to almost anything in and of itself can be framed as a health problem. Second, gambling addiction may have negative effects on one's resources and personal relations. Third, excessive machine use may have direct negative effects on the body itself, especially one's mental health. Framed as a health problem, video poker addiction can then elicit a variety of health care responses, from twelve-step programs to interventions by health professionals. These responses can themselves be a form of medical consumption, shaped by the perceived needs of the addicted as well as the actions of the promoters of different programs, health care professionals, and third-party payers.

Within Western industrialized societies, "addiction" and other diseases of consumption often follow a pattern of initial association with the relatively more affluent (who often start trends, are the initial target market, and have resources to spend), followed by greater prevalence among poorer people. And even when consumption is equally distributed, the negative impact of technologies is often experienced unequally by people with fewer resources. A recent newspaper report called attention to the fact that well-intentioned efforts to narrow the digital divide between rich and poor in the U.S. had unintended consequences. The gap has indeed narrowed, but poorer people are apparently using their connectivity to do more wasteful things with their time. They reportedly watch television shows and videos, play games, and connect on social networking sites much more than richer people. "This growing time-wasting gap, policy makers and researchers say, is more a reflection of the ability of parents to monitor and limit how children use technology than of access to it."[8] Not only do economic, cultural, and social differences mediate the way new commodities and technologies are understood and consumed, but what types and patterns of consumption are labeled as health risks and stigmatized (with resulting "looping" impacts on behavior) may be influenced by the interests of particular groups.[9]

What I want to call attention to here is the interaction between the culturally specific intelligent design and marketing of consumer goods and the coincident framing of addiction and excessive consumption as a disease, which may itself elicit consumer-oriented health-restoring responses. I imagine the perplexed early twenty-first-century Martian arriving at her motel room in the U.S. after her long trip and turning on the television. How would she make sense of the marketing of calorie-dense, super-sized, highly processed food stuffs along with the direct-to-consumer medical advertisements pitching heart disease risk–reducing medicines as well as commercials for weight loss programs, gym memberships, and exercise machines?

This pattern repeats itself in other types of consumption and societal response, and leads to a more expansive and complicated conception of what is commonly referred to as risks or diseases of affluence or civilization. It is no longer adequate to attribute these problems to evolutionary models of "cave men in the fast lane" and to the changed material conditions of modern life.[10] The ill health associated with affluence does not simply result from environmental dangers like radon or collateral damage from economic development. It is also a matter of why certain patterns of consumption take root and are understood as health risks.

Consider the increasing attention given to the health consequences associated with obesity such as diabetes, heart disease, disability, and premature death. It has also been noted that in the United States, as in some other industrialized countries, obesity is more prevalent among the poor and the stigmatized minorities. Almost all attention to explaining and responding to this disparity centers on the putative beliefs, economic conditions, and neighborhood characteristics that impact diet and physical activity. But obesity as medicalized risk can also be understood in dynamic social terms, and in ways that have little to do with the material determinants of diet and physical activity. Let me explain via an analogy to socially patterned linguistic variation.

Postvowel "r-dropping" (not articulating the r sound in words like car or card) was once a distinctive feature of upper-class speech in some American communities. As a marker of prestige, it was later adopted by the lower classes. But upper-class speakers gradually added the r back as r-dropping became the norm for lower social classes. This dynamic is an example of a much needed and socially constructed difference or disparity. Linguist William Labov conducted an experiment in three New York City department stores in the 1960s that showed how the social stratification of r-dropping had stabilized while suggesting that immediate social context also played a role. Salespersons in more prestigious stores pronounced the postvowel rs much more than salespersons in less prestigious stores. But salespersons in less prestigious stores tended to pronounce the r more when they were made to feel self-conscious, such as when the experimenter asked departments store workers to repeat the answer to a question about which floor (i.e., fourth) a certain piece of merchandise might be found on.[11]

A dynamic similar to such sociolinguistic variation may lie behind the formation and persistence of many consumption-based health disparities. In both the social patterning of language and health, difference or disparity may largely function to signal and maintain class and other social distinctions.[12] Some health disparities and gradients may not result from other social inequalities in any direct sense but serve rather as markers of class, wealth, and/or race. These disparities, in other words, are purposeful and functional in themselves even if there is no single person or group of people consciously plotting things out.

Some or a large amount of the social patterning of obesity may be an instance of this kind of framing phenomenon rather than being caused solely by differences in diets, the built environment of inner cities, and the marketing of obesogenic foods to particular groups (e.g., McDonald's branding as an African American foodstuff).[13] Some of the ethnic/racial and socioeconomic disparity evident in obesity rates may be functional, a direct by-product of fundamental social dynamics, especially important in explaining the enthusiasm for the current medicalization of obesity as a health risk and the class-tinged decisions made by individuals. Like r-dropping, higher average weight historically (in an era of more expensive calories) was more prevalent among the better off. It also took on some symbolic value as a marker of socioeconomic progress and advancement. But as cheap calories became more widely available, the poor gained weight. What was once a marker of high socioeconomic standing lost its meaning, and the social dynamic of differentiation meant that many who had the resources to reduce their weight or evade obesity did so. Supporting this dynamic has been an economy of nonconsumption as a commodity — low-fat foods, gyms, etc. — in which there has been more and easier participation by affluent people.

In other words, obesity has become a marker for lower prestige and status in society. People with greater resources have more ability to avoid the stigma of obesity. The enthusiasm with which obesity has been framed as a public health threat and risk factor has allowed the better off to put additional distance between them and those less fortunate. Thus one can even view the medicalization of overweight and perhaps moderate obesity, constituted as a risk state, as a framing mechanism for signaling and maintaining social difference. In our secular society that enshrines health as a transcendent value, there may be no better way to stigmatize certain groups or classes than to associate a real or perceived difference from others with a bad health outcome. These are macro-level determinants that do not have to be consciously uttered and negotiated. Rather, like *r*-dropping, there is something preconscious about them. But one would miss the dynamic that maintains and fuels the "disparity" if we thought of weight gain by different social groups as simply the result of material conditions in which groups lived and their unique histories, values, and cultures. Interactions among disease classifications, social dynamics, and differential access to resources might explain the appearance and persistence of disparities in obesity and other health risks. And these within-country class dynamics can appear to be reproducing themselves in the relations between rich and poor countries and regions of the world (chapter 8).

IV

Throughout these chapters, I mostly focus on the clinical and public health origins and consequences of *risky medicine*. But these developments are at the same time tied to broader social, cultural, and economic factors within American society and elsewhere. They have been shaped, for example, by excess risk intervention capacity in developed countries (chapter 8) and demands for increased surveillance and threat assessment post-9/11. They also reflect the values and interests of the societies from which they emerged. The enthusiasm for some risk interventions, e.g., some cancer screening tests and diet-cancer associations, seems to me to partly represent a form of death denial. Compliance with screening regimens or cancer prevention diets can give Americans the illusion of warding off the inevitable and controlling the uncontrollable.

The priority given to medicalized, individual-centered risk reduction also has its origins in a self-sustaining feedback loop that is manifested in other aspects of social life such as schooling, personal safety, and Social Security. In these domains, the commitments made to individual- rather than societal-level remedies are often self-reinforcing. People have greater reason to choose individual solutions when there is little faith in the efficacy or reliability of collective action, while the choice itself may increase the perception and reality that there is little security provided by society, further undermining collective action. Reduced support or threatened reductions in Social Security can drive individuals to make more individualized solutions to retirement planning, which may itself, via reduced expectations of need, lead to reduced political support for Social Security taxes. The political will to fund defined benefits for city and state employees has been similarly undermined by the decades-long shift to private, self-directed retirement plans in the private sector. Similar dynamics can occur when more individuals choose private over public schooling or attempt to control crime by living in gated communities rather than adopting safety measures within regions that include both poor and rich areas.

In a similar way, the consequences of *risky medicine* potentially reach far beyond the clinic and the individual patient/consumer. Due to limited resources, intellectual bandwidth, and imagination, the individual-centered high-risk approach to disease prevention can crowd out more broad-based society-level approaches.[14] Pharmacological agents for tobacco addiction may have greater appeal than constraining tobacco production and marketing because they target the individual with a problem, resemble and can be readily incorporated into a typical clinical encounter, and seem high-tech and scientific.

It is not surprising that there may be considerable NIH and industry funding of research into these agents while the health consequences of social and economic policies are usually not even understood as health interventions.

The developments explored in this book, especially the shift in medical and lay attention from symptomatic illness to risk states and the converged experience of risk and disease, have also led to some flattening of the idiosyncrasy that is characteristic of symptom-initiated medical encounters. Individuals recruited into high-risk groups by screening tests are often more easily categorized and counted and generally have more uniform experiences than people suffering symptomatic disease. Identifying and treating someone in a high-risk category is often much less messy than diagnosing and treating people with pain, fatigue, and organ dysfunction. This more uniform, externally visible, and quantifiable experience, along with more commonly shared decisions and interventions, has gradually taken up a larger fraction of medical encounters and expenditures (chapter 2).

These developments, not surprisingly, permit more external evaluation of the quality and cost of medical care because more people can be seen as suffering the same or similar problem, and the details of their experiences are more readily visualized and counted. The management of expectant consequences in someone at risk for disease complications on the basis of "early" diagnosis and membership in a risk state is often more legible, visible, and uniform than diagnosing and treating symptomatic disease. People with abnormal screening lipid tests, "early" good-prognosis cancer or precancer, hypertension, prediabetes, etc. often are otherwise healthy and start their diagnostic career from a similar baseline, from which they can be compared to people in other settings or exposed to different interventions.

Because of this visibility and uniformity, government and third-party payers commonly employ compliance with guidelines of risk reduction practices and products as quality indicators, e.g., whether aspirin or beta blockers are prescribed after heart attacks (a well-established means of secondary prevention in heart disease), how many people of a certain age are screened for high cholesterol, etc. Health systems and practices can be measured for their compliance with these measures and be financially rewarded or punished. Individual patients' compliance can be similarly surveyed and measured.

There are obvious downsides to these practices. Just because risks and risk interventions are more uniform and more visible for auditing does not mean they are important indicators of health or health care quality. The situation is analogous to the oft-told story of the person who is looking for his keys under a lamppost on the opposite side of the street from where he lost them because the light is better there.

The transformations described in *Risky Medicine* thus bring with them the potential for more state and corporate control over individual medical decisions and patienthood. Because there is more order and visibility in many risk states than exists among people with symptomatic disease, there is more opportunity for state and third-party evaluation and management. This can facilitate schemes to monitor individuals and populations for health gains which may serve more political than health ends, be appealing and commonsensical, but wasteful.[15] Like teachers who respond to incentives to reward better outcomes by teaching to the test, physicians and patients may waste time and resources carrying out and documenting compliance with marginally effective or ineffective screening tests, preventive medications, and counseling for lifestyle change.

Because of these medical, economic, social, and political implications, there is an evident need to recover some of the choices made on the road to *risky medicine* and the nature and extent of the resulting transformation of American medicine and the illness experience.

2

The converged experience
of risk and disease

As a second-year medical student three decades ago, I watched a senior physician approach one house officer after another asking for the names of hospitalized patients on whom students could practice taking medical histories and performing physical examinations. A suitable patient would have been admitted to the hospital with an as yet undiagnosed collection of symptoms and signs (in addition to being conscious and able to speak English). Each house officer was in charge of thirty to fifty patients but could find only one or two who were suitable.

My medical teachers had evoked in their lectures and at the bedside the sick patient who experienced illness uncorrupted by medical knowledge and prior medical intervention. That few such patients existed in the hospital did little damage to this ideal type, whose existence was sustained by older assumptions about clinical practice and medical education.

In the intervening years, the gap between our idealized view of the sick patient and the actual one who attends our hospitals and clinics has only grown. Hospital and outpatient care is less often about new, undiagnosed, symptomatic problems than it is about existing chronic disease, especially the expectant management of problems predicted or found by other interventions and earlier medical surveillance, for example, the placement of pacemakers in patients previously found to have slow or irregular heartbeats or colonoscopies done after an abnormal fecal occult blood test.

Central to patients' actual presenting complaints has been a new risk-dominated way of experiencing health and disease. While many observers have noted medicine's increasing focus on disease prevention and risk among the erstwhile healthy, few have recognized the profound parallel developments among the already sick or diagnosed.

Some observers have highlighted the important role of the pharmaceutical industry and medical research in jointly producing both new preventive medicines and the new risk factors that these medicines target.[1] Others have stressed a new style of medical surveillance in which normal populations have been surveyed and subjected to a growing number of demands to comply with medical directives.[2] Although these accounts focus on the radical expansion of preventive medicine into the otherwise healthy population, much less attention has been paid to parallel developments among the chronically ill. There has been a profound, if largely unnoticed, shift in who is understood to be suffering from chronic disease and the disease experience itself. In many instances, chronic disease has become a kind of risk state in which diagnosis, treatment, and "disease management" are directed not at relieving symptoms but at reducing the chances of anticipated, feared developments.

This shift has resulted in a converged experience of risk and chronic disease. On one side of this convergence, the number of otherwise healthy individuals who are considered to be "at risk for," or have risk factors for, a particular disease has grown immensely; their bodies have been subjected to increased surveillance; and the risk state itself has become more embodied and, in other ways, more disease-like. In large measure, these changes have resulted from the expanding medicalization processes noted by sociologists and others over the past few decades. From the other side, the experience of chronic disease increasingly resembles the experience of people at risk for disease.

Distinguishing the disease experience from the risk experience is difficult because so many developments are obliterating this difference. In everyday usage, *disease* is understood to be a pathological process producing ill health, including symptoms. The *risk* of disease is some statistical probability that ill health might happen. As an imminent state, there can be no illness experience that emanates *from* risk in any direct, physiological sense (of course, emotional distress and other psychological consequences often follow from knowledge of and beliefs about risk).[3] If readers are imagining exceptions to these definitions, they are probably thinking about the processes I am describing. Screening and early detection of HIV, for example, can, in a very short time, transform someone from feeling healthy to being "positive for HIV," leading to preventive drug treatments that cause symptoms.

I do not want to leave the impression that the changes that result in this convergence are solely the result of developments within medical practice and biomedical knowledge production, although these are my main foci. Sociologists and others have observed that Western societies are increasingly becoming *risk societies*. Such societies engage in the politics of risk distribution as much as resource allocation, are facing dangers of borderless and often invisible global threats (bird flu, terrorism, extensively resistant tuberculosis, global warming), and thus are turning inward—reflexively—to make sense of these dangers and responses.[4] Although we should be wary of the flattening of nuance and detail that can follow from such broad frameworks, it is worth underscoring that the developments explored below share with the *risk society* theoretical framework the emphasis that both risks and the societal responses they elicit have technological origins.

What is the converged experience of chronic disease and risk?

Imagine two women, one who is suffering from breast cancer and the second "merely" at risk for the disease. The first woman is fifty-eight years old. Two years earlier, she detected a lump in her left breast. After an aspiration biopsy revealed cancerous cells, she had a lumpectomy and removal of lymph nodes in her armpit (none of which contained cancer), followed by a course of local radiation and then six months of chemotherapy. After this acute treatment, she was put on a five-year course of the "antiestrogen" Tamoxifen. She now closely follows developments in breast cancer. At the moment, she is concerned about whether to start another kind of hormonal therapy after her course of Tamoxifen ends and whether she should begin getting screening breast MRIs and/or more frequent mammography. For these and other questions, she frequently searches the web and attends meetings of breast cancer survivor and advocacy groups.

The second woman also is fifty-eight years old. She took birth control pills during her twenties, had her first child at age thirty-four, and, at the urging of her gynecologist, took supplementary estrogen pills starting at age fifty because of menopausal symptoms and to prevent heart disease and osteoporosis. A few years later her doctor told her to stop taking these pills because new medical evidence had conclusively shown that their risks—especially an increased risk of developing breast cancer—outweighed their putative benefits. Since age forty, she has been getting annual mammograms. Four years ago, she had an abnormal mammogram, which led to an aspiration biopsy that did not show cancer. Fearful of developing breast cancer, she is attentive to media reports and periodically browses the Internet for new information on cancer prevention. She has seen direct-to-consumer advertisements for Tamoxifen as a preventive measure for women at high risk of breast cancer. She understands that she has multiple risk factors for breast cancer, such as being postmenopausal, having had her first child after thirty, having earlier used hormone replacement therapy, and having a history of a benign breast biopsy. She has sought advice from friends, doctors, and breast cancer advocacy groups about whether to take Tamoxifen and/or to find other means of reducing her risk of breast cancer.

At present, the first woman does not experience any symptoms of cancer but nonetheless undergoes intensive surveillance, has concerns about the long-term effects of previous treatments, and faces the future with caution. The experience of the second women is not very different. She may well decide to take Tamoxifen to prevent breast cancer. Like the first woman, she undergoes frequent surveillance and faces the future with caution. Both women face an array of similar choices and seek guidance in similar places. They share fears for the future, feelings of randomness and uncertainty, and pressures for self-surveillance. Both seek ways to regain a sense of control and face difficult decisions about preventive treatment and consumption. They are part of a larger breast cancer risk-to-disease continuum which includes scientists' understanding of the disease and which has resulted in a large, mobilized group for advocacy, fund raising, and awareness.[5]

What has made chronic disease more risky?

That the major causes of morbidity and mortality have shifted over the past two centuries from acute to chronic disease is both a historical and an epidemiological truism. Yet not as obvious has been the way in which the management of risk has become a central feature of the disease experience. How has the chronic disease experience become so dominated by risk?

I suggest five reasons: (1) new clinical interventions that have directly changed the natural history of disease; (2) greater biological, clinical, and epidemiological knowledge of chronic disease risk; (3) recruitment of larger numbers of people into chronic disease diagnoses through new screening and diagnostic technology and disease definitions; (4) new ways of conceptualizing efficacy of risk-reducing products and practices; and (5) intense diagnostic testing and medical intervention.

*Clinical interventions that have directly changed
the natural history of disease*

Beginning in the early twentieth century, scientists and clinicians developed new interventions that removed or alleviated signs and symptoms of acute pathological processes but did not entirely eradicate the underlying chronic disease. These interventions transformed the patients' experience of their disease. Perhaps the most dramatic and earliest example was the transformative role of insulin on the diabetes experience.[6] Insulin treatment gave doctors and patients a way to control hyperglycemia. For many children with type 1 diabetes, life spans changed from a few months or years after diagnosis to many decades. At the same time, however, the insulin treatment itself did not simply substitute for the normal operations of the diseased pancreas. It produced its own life-threatening problems, required constant monitoring and decision making, and often became an arena of conflict over control and responsibility among children, parents, and their doctors. Moreover, by allowing diabetics to avoid diabetic coma and live with their disease for decades, insulin therapy uncovered a host of more difficult-to-manage and largely hidden metabolic and other abnormalities that diabetes produces, including damage to the kidney, heart, nerves, and eyes.

The disease experience was similarly transformed for breast cancer at the beginning of the twentieth century.[7] Surgical innovators like William Halsted promoted radical cancer surgery, and life after radical surgery was often very different from the breast cancer experience of earlier eras. Many women no longer suffered from growing and recurring tumors in their chest. In the absence of detectable "external" disease and after punishing treatment with often severe side effects, they often believed that their suffering bought them a greater chance of survival. But the radical surgery did not appreciably change patients' ultimate prognosis. Halsted understood this incomplete and frustrating reality, reluctantly acknowledging that radical surgery had little effect on the late metastatic stage of cancer's natural history, which was responsible for its deadliness. Indeed, Halsted generally avoided discussing with his patients the possibility of future metastatic disease until he was forced to when the cancer recurred.

Even though Halsted encouraged his breast cancer patients to get on with their lives after radical surgery and keep a stiff upper lip, they did not generally follow this advice. Postmastectomy patients were understandably fearful that their cancer would return and sought reassurance and examinations by physicians, surveyed their bodies, and wondered about steps they could take to prevent future disease. Many women believed their cancer surgery had been effective because their attentiveness to changes in their bodies had led them to seek medical attention in the nick of time. After surgery, many understandably surveyed their own bodies systematically and wanted frequent checkups.

During this same period, new medical interventions such as radiation and radium therapy were developed to deal with recurring cancer. Although these treatments were unlikely to cure the cancer, their high scientific status and powerful effects led many patients to believe in their efficacy and strengthened their vigilance to catch cancer recurrences in time for these treatments to succeed. In sum, many of these early twentieth-century patients after surgery lived a "life at risk," one filled with fear, close surveillance of their bodies, and increased demand for medical examinations. They hungered for some means to reassert control over their fears that their cancer would return. At the end of their lives, patients with recurrences also experienced a highly intervened-in last stage of illness.

The breast cancer experience, like the experience of many diabetes patients, had been transformed. Unlike diabetes but perhaps more like the majority of other twentieth-century diseases subject to new medical treatments, this transformation was due to many indirect and collateral effects of new treatments as well as to the direct effects on the natural history of disease.

Increased biological, clinical, and epidemiological
knowledge of chronic disease risk

A key driver of the risk-centered chronic disease experience has been the explosion in knowledge, such as new details and models of the natural history of disease, associations among laboratory, radiological, and other test findings and disease etiology and prognosis, new frameworks for understanding disease, and molecular and other insights into disease mechanisms. As a result of clinical and epidemiological study, for example, we have learned that patients with inflammatory bowel disease have an increased risk of colon cancer. Knowledge of this increased risk has led to efforts at the secondary prevention of cancer (*secondary prevention* means the early detection of disease or other efforts to ward off the harmful effects of disease progression, and *primary prevention* implies efforts to avoid the disease in the first place). Almost all inflammatory bowel disease patients are urged to get annual colonoscopies and sometimes to get prophylactic surgery.

Clinical and epidemiological study and intense diagnostic testing have combined to create a web of knowledge in which the variation in any number of laboratory tests and physiological parameters is associated with a higher risk of some untoward outcome. Increasingly, having one disease puts you at risk for another. For example, so-called routine diagnostic blood testing may uncover a high serum protein level. This will lead to more sophisticated and expensive testing to determine the exact nature of the protein and may ultimately lead to a diagnosis of a monoclonal gammopathy, which is an abnormal pattern of antibody production that does not itself produce symptoms and occurs in 2 to 4 percent of adults over fifty. Through epidemiological, clinical, and laboratory studies, however, we have come to understand this condition as part of a continuum of abnormalities that include a cancer called multiple myeloma. An individual found to have a monoclonal gammopathy is typically counseled there is some small annual risk, perhaps 1 chance in a hundred, of developing multiple myeloma, so he or she understandably enters into a world of concern about the future and close surveillance so that interventions against this cancer may be deployed early (although the decision about when to initiate treatment is complex).

Each year, other entirely new conditions are created based on observations of potential clinical outcomes following abnormal tests performed in the course of routine medical care and screening. To take another example, the antiphospholipid antibody syndrome is a set of potential complications that are associated with this antibody, which is itself often detected because of other incidental abnormalities (which clinicians ironically label incidentalomas as their clinical significance is often unclear). In the case of antiphospholipid antibodies, their measurement is often triggered by an abnormal clotting time or false positive syphilis test discovered during the evaluation or monitoring of some other problem.

A greater knowledge of the risks associated with existing or new diagnoses understandably leads to difficult choices and uncertainties. After being tested in routine laboratory tests or before donating blood, millions of Americans have learned that they have silent hepatitis C infection.[8] Clinical and epidemiological studies have revealed that hepatitis C infection is likely to remain asymptomatic but that some of those infected will later develop serious and possibly fatal chronic liver disease. There have been many attempts to reach a consensus on how to deal with this uncertainty, including the risk posed to others. Should the general population be screened? Among those with serological evidence of infection, who should have more advanced tests and procedures (including liver biopsy) which might help with decisions, themselves fraught with uncertainty, about who should be treated with costly and dangerous medicines such as interferon and ribavirin.[9]

We are only at the beginning of the road to new and redefined diseases leading from the exponential rise in correlations between variations in the human genome and various states of health and disease and the likely profound impact on the risk experience.[10] The result will likely be more people who are aware for longer periods of time about possible future ill health and who will be advised to modify their lifestyle and undergo different types of surveillance and preventive medical treatment.

Changes in screening, diagnostic technologies, and disease
definitions lead to more convergence

Larger numbers of people are having a risk-dominated chronic disease experience because of the creation and diffusion of increasingly sensitive screening technologies, "earlier" definitions of pathological states, and lowered thresholds for clinical diagnosis. In some diseases, such as breast cancer, "early" diagnosis, often picked up by more sensitive screening tests (such as the recent use of MRIs to screen for breast cancer), has grown almost independently of any change in the numbers of women with recurrent and often fatal disease. In such cases, I would argue that the increased numbers of people who experience this risk-centered chronic disease are an *addition to* the people who experience disease in older ways rather than an *exchange of* one characteristic disease experience for another, such as occurred in type 1 diabetes mellitus in the early twentieth century.

Increased numbers of people have a risk-centered chronic disease experience because of new disease categories that are constructed as "earlier" and less prototypical presentations of existing diseases. Peter Kramer, for example, has argued for such *formes frustes* psychiatric diagnoses, like low self-esteem, chronic minor depression, social inhibition, and anhedonia.[11] Much of this *diagnosis creep* is driven by pharmaceutical companies that want to expand markets for their products in league with physicians and other moral entrepreneurs who champion the expanded disease categories.

There are many examples of other new *predisease* states that result from enlarging the catchment area of existing categories to include "earlier" points in a disease's natural history. Defined by pathologists but sustained by screening campaigns, different cervical and breast precancers have been discovered and widely diagnosed throughout the latter half of the twentieth century. Breast cancer has had an exponential growth of precancers, largely driven by the widespread use of screening mammography. The incidence of lobular and ductal carcinoma in situ, for example, jumped from a rate of 11.3 per 100,000 women per year in 1975 to an astounding 91.2 per 100,000 women in 2002.[12]

Each year, more than 3 million American women are found to have a Pap smear abnormality, typically ASCUS (atypical squamous cells of uncertain significance). ASCUS is part of a continuum of "precancerous" abnormalities that have constantly been redefined and reclassified over the past decades. As a result, women with this very common abnormality enter a continuum of risk, which often requires more frequent surveillance and more invasive diagnostic procedures.

Prehypertension and prediabetes are, in some ways, simpler phenomena. They are defined by lower thresholds along the same continuous axis—blood pressure and serum glucose, respectively—that have been used to define the fully formed disease states. Hypertension, I should note, is itself an asymptomatic risk factor for heart disease and stroke. But its long history, objective definition, and medical treatment have given it a borderline disease status in common medical usage and practice.

The experience of people diagnosed with the different precancers, prehypertension, and prediabetes can be very similar to that of people with cancer, hypertension, and type 2 diabetes. In hypertension and type 2 diabetes, the medical treatment for both the disease and the predisease diagnosis and treatment can be almost identical, as is the *risky* meaning of the diagnosis for recruited individuals. In most cases, members of the original disease, like the new predisease group, do not suffer symptoms referable to the disease. It also should not be surprising that the resulting larger group of people attached to the diabetes or hypertension class of diseases coalesce into one large market for new preventive drugs and other interventions.[13]

New ways of conceptualizing efficacy

As I will discuss in much greater detail in the next chapter, the emergence of at-risk chronic disease is predicated on highly subjective ways of evaluating efficacy. For example, individual compliance with screening and diagnostic tests, a prerequisite for recruiting individuals into risk states, depends on the individual's judgment that these tests "work." Throughout the twentieth century, men and women wrestled with different disease prevention messages, such as the one to examine the body for dangerous signs of cancer and to seek medical treatment without delay if something suspicious is found. Later in the century, similar individual decisions about efficacy had to be made about cancer screening programs like Pap smears and mammography. In both these cases, efficacy was often understood in highly individual and psychological terms, in addition to medical and lay perceptions of their scientific efficacy based on absent or contested data. These early detection and screening programs largely "worked" by giving individuals a way to assert some control over their fears of cancer.[14]

Such social efficacy calculations also help explain data suggesting that many Americans today who have experienced false positive cancer screening tests generally do not feel harmed or become skeptical of the screening enterprise. Instead, they typically feel more invested in the screening paradigm. One interpretation is that being given a cancer diagnosis and then having it taken away is experienced as a victory over cancer, leading to a greater sense of control over cancer and fears of cancer.[15]

Risk-reducing pharmaceuticals similarly promise to eliminate or control the fears, discomfort, and hassles associated with risk. This rationale is not often trumpeted and, if made explicit, is combined with more objective claims of efficacy against disease.

Whether asserting control over fear or for other purposes, we have become accustomed to accepting the efficacy of many interventions as reducing the probability of this or that bad outcome. In the last years of his life, my father suffered from memory loss, confusion, and disorientation. Fearful that he would hurt himself and others, we sent him to a clinic that specialized in evaluating mental decline among the elderly. After a series of neuropsychological and radiological evaluations, he was diagnosed with Alzheimer's disease, told to stop driving, and prescribed Aricept. Obtaining a diagnosis and a prescription is the expected outcome of a medical encounter, but it obscures the historically new prominence of the risk calculus lying behind so many decisions in chronic disease. Like so many other drugs for chronic disease aimed at positively influencing the natural history of the disease, evidence from clinical trials of Aricept showed some statistically significant advantage in symptoms for people taking the drug. Nobody's Alzheimer's disease got better; rather, the rate of decline was, on average, less steep for people taking the medicine than for those taking a placebo. The individual taking Aricept would never experience efficacy in the way that a person taking a pain reliever, a curative cancer treatment, or an antibiotic that led to symptom improvement would. Instead, efficacy is a promise of a positive deviation from a projected downhill trajectory. This kind of efficacy calculus has become commonplace and has eased the acceptance of many risk interventions and the risk states they target.

Intense diagnostic testing and treatment

Finally, the chronic disease experience has become more risk centered because of the intensity of modern medical intervention, both diagnostic and therapeutic. Increased diagnostic testing in the course of caring for patients has led to an ever-expanding web of putative associations between different objective markers of clinical variation (blood tests, X-rays, etc.) and the probabilities of different diseases. Residents and interns in American hospitals used to walk around in white coats weighted down with manuals and crib sheets that contain lists of possible outcomes of every conceivable abnormal blood test, X-ray, EKG pattern, urine test, and the like—today they are more likely to find such information, the magnitude of which has only grown, from their smart phones. This intense testing contributes to the web of knowledge discussed earlier and also is the entry point for the *career* of the patient with the newly discovered abnormality.[16]

The parallel role of therapeutic interventions is illustrated by the creation of an entirely new major category of disease experience, that of cancer survivorship, the subject of chapter 7. Cancer has long been understood and experienced as an encounter with increasing dangers to health, culminating in pain, wasting, and death. As such, it has been both greatly feared and subject to medical and popular routines aimed at evading this or that outcome. In these respects, it is the ultimate risky disease, putting patient and doctor in real and potential conflict with an enfolding, devastating narrative. Over the past decades, with a generation of cancer survivors outliving the immediate threat of the disease, knowledge of the risks throughout one's lifetime—emanating from both the natural history of cancer and different modalities of treatment—has exploded. The dimensions of this transformation are huge, in part because the numbers of people who constitute the class of cancer survivors is growing. According to government estimates, the number of "cancer survivors" rose from slightly more than 2 million in 1971 to more than 10 million in 2003.[17] In one sense, cancer survivorship is the kind of direct and successful consequence of intervening in the natural history of disease discussed earlier in the transformation of type 1 diabetes. But in other ways, cancer survivorship has been dominated by the possible long-term consequences of treatment as much as, or more than, by the transformed disease itself.

It is not surprising that a compendium of evidence-based guidelines for the long-term follow-up of children previously treated for cancer was 179 pages long. Experts recommend, for example, that children who received anthracycline antibiotics (a common chemotherapy class that includes drugs such as doxorubicin) should have yearly blood counts, baseline and then periodic EKGs, echocardiograms, or heart nuclear scans, and counseling regarding appropriate weight, blood pressure, diet, and exercise.[18] A medical textbook devoted entirely to medical surveillance after cancer treatment contains 106 chapters. Despite the extensive review of known complications from surgery, radiation, chemotherapy, and the lingering effects of the cancer itself, the authors bemoan the poor evidence base for many of the most commonly used surveillance regimes (say PSA surveillance post-treatment for prostate cancer).[19]

Similar surveillance for serious late effects from cancer treatment follows from knowledge that chemotherapy and radiation can cause endocrine dysfunction (e.g., adrenal insufficiency from cranial radiation), neurological disorders (e.g., neuropathy), lung disease, kidney disease, and hearing problems. Perhaps most feared are new cancers caused by earlier cancer treatment. In addition to these mechanisms, transfusions often given during treatment may lead to chronic infectious disease (e.g., hepatitis C in the era before screening), and steroids may lead to cataracts and other sequelae. Survival itself puts people at risk of delayed and/or chronic psychiatric disorders, especially depression. Recommendations to screen and watch for all these late complications create a formidable challenge to the care and peace of mind of cancer survivors—all in addition to fears of and actions to be taken to survey the body for and ultimately prevent or treat early any recurrence of the original cancer.

For many people who experience other highly intervened-in chronic diseases that are not as deadly as untreated cancer but that require constant treatment, the risks associated with medications mean worry, screening, and lifestyle modification. Today, many patients with severe rheumatoid arthritis take drugs like Plaquenil, Methotrexate, and Enbrel to influence positively the natural history of disease. Plaquenil is an antimalarial drug that is believed to have a modifying effect on the disease. Unfortunately, there is a much-feared rare side effect of retinal damage. Out of concern for this complication, patients are told to get baseline and routine examinations by an ophthalmologist. Methotrexate is a folate antagonist often used as a chemotherapeutic agent against cancer. It also is believed to have a disease-modifying effect on rheumatoid arthritis. Among other side effects, it can be toxic to the liver. Because of that, doctors frequently order liver function blood tests and warn patients to not drink alcohol excessively or to do anything else that might further compromise the liver. Enbrel is a highly innovative recombinant DNA product containing two immunologically active proteins. Unfortunately, the same immune-modifying effect that helps stabilize or modify an autoimmune disease process like rheumatoid arthritis also can modify the host's immune response to infection, making patients especially vulnerable to some infectious diseases. As a result, patients are told to stop Enbrel at the first sign of an infectious disease, to take special precautions to avoid infection, and to start antibiotics if they develop a cough, fever, or other symptom of infection. An increased risk of cancer has been reported associated with the general class of immune-modifying drugs used to modulate the course of chronic inflammatory conditions like rheumatoid arthritis, greatly adding to this already highly *risky* chronic disease experience.[20]

Consequences and implications

The transformed chronic disease experience and its convergence with the growing numbers of people recruited into risk states have contributed to a great deal of improvement in individual and population health, for example, the dramatic survival benefits of insulin treatment for children with type 1 diabetes mellitus and the role played by the diabetes risk continuum in rationalizing some public health efforts against childhood obesity. At the same time, some unsettling and generally underappreciated consequences might be subjected to more clinical and policy reflection and response.

Chronic disease today entails a great deal of expectant treatment and surveillance for other diseases and complications. Physicians routinely prescribe inhaled steroids to prevent asthma exacerbations and lipid-lowering drugs, beta blockers, and aspirin to prevent a second heart attack. Belief in the efficacy of such secondary prevention at the same time serves as an incentive to make more and earlier diagnoses of the condition that is the object of secondary prevention efforts. For example, belief in the efficacy of early intervention drives the earlier diagnosis of childhood autism and the growing number of children diagnosed with Asperger's syndrome. While individual clinicians and families might understandably have a very low threshold to accept evidence of the efficacy of early behavioral interventions for autism— the putative benefits seem plausible while the risks appear low—this acceptance at the same time can in aggregate drive the broadening of the disease's definition and the increase in numbers diagnosed, which may be less of a good thing. This interaction between belief in the efficacy of secondary prevention and the expansion of disease diagnoses and the changed character of the chronic disease experience has not been widely appreciated and represents an opportunity for novel policy analysis and intervention (as elaborated in chapter 9).

The intensity of testing, anticipatory, or expectant treatment and the belief that such maneuvering is consequential have led to greater efforts at *disease management*. The idea is that there are enough predictive tests, preventive maneuvers, surveillance, and other routines tied to specific conditions that management systems—case workers, patient education materials, reminder systems—will keep patients healthier and reduce costs, especially by avoided or deferred hospital admissions. These elements constitute the career of the bureaucratic patient.[21]

In asthma, for example, patients have been urged to develop "action plans" in cooperation with their doctors that specify detailed, individualized plans for adjusting medications and seeking medical care in response to changes in symptoms, signs, and home techni-cal monitoring (e.g., spirometry). Such plans also list environmental and other individual triggers of asthma exacerbations. Such detailed, explicit management can profoundly change the asthma experience. Among other effects, they increase the nodal points at which the clini-cal situation needs to be assessed and management decisions must be made.

For many patients, the experience of chronic disease is not domi-nated by symptoms of the pathological processes but by reading the body for signs of future problems, negotiating different secondary prevention measures, and making decisions about the future. Many people with no symptoms are diagnosed with type 2 diabetes melli-tus because of laboratory abnormalities alone. Many other patients with symptoms of excessive thirst and urination will become asymp-tomatic soon after diagnosis and the beginnings of lifestyle change and/or medical treatment. But asymptomatic does not mean that they have no *experience* of disease. Patients will understand that they are at higher risk of heart disease and will need to be screened ag-gressively for known heart disease risk factors. They are likely to pay special attention to any chest pains as potential angina pectoris. They are not only urged to get nutritional counseling and diabetes educa-tion but are also likely to be screened regularly for different diabetes complications: kidney disease, eye problems, and so forth. If they are prescribed with medications, they need to watch out for side effects—especially hypoglycemia—that need monitoring and attention. Many new medicines and interventions are reported in the health and business pages of daily newspapers and on local and national news. Patients closely follow the significant media coverage of the many controversies over efficacy and the inevitable side effects that follow from mass use and study.

As a growing fraction of the chronic disease experience becomes secondary prevention and surveillance rather than the experience of symptoms, and more of the disease population is asymptomatic or minimally symptomatic from the disease itself, the disease experience also becomes more uniform, and thus an individual's illness experi-ence becomes more legible to third parties and others. These trans-formations rationalize and permit more external control of decision making such as practice guidelines and protocols. Explicit evidence-based evaluation of particular products and practices, an important and necessary policy response, often means less attention to aspects of the disease experience that are not uniform or predictable enough to be managed by protocols and in standard ways. Given the limits of our interest and material resources, we focus on what is legible and measurable, for example, measuring the hemoglobin A1C rates of diabetes patients (which roughly correlate with sugar control over weeks or months) or the prescription of secondary preventive asthma medications as measures of quality of care, rewarding and punishing providers and health systems on the basis of their compliance with these measures, but ignoring less legible but consequential idiosyncratic practices and outcomes.

The convergence of risk and disease has had more subtle effects on individual decision making, important to the individuals involved, but also having widespread effects. There has been an understandable expansion of decision-making patterns or styles routinely used by people with symptomatic, serious disease to individuals whose illness experience falls at different points on the risk continuum. For example, some women with metastatic breast cancer have opted for treatments that medical evidence suggests are not in aggregate beneficial, like the use of highly toxic chemotherapy followed by bone marrow transplant. Faced with the near certainty of advancing disease and death, it is understandable that some women choose to bet against the odds, hoping their one roll of the dice will lead to survival. They may also want to avoid regretting later that they did not do everything possible to avert advancing disease and death.

These "playing by the law of small numbers" and "anticipated regret" heuristics have become increasingly operative in decisions about risk.[22] For example, some women and doctors invoke these heuristics to explain their support for screening mammography for women under fifty, despite data indicating no or minimal overall benefit and considerable financial and personal costs. They fear cancer so much that gambling against the odds seems reasonable. Women may also anticipate the regret they would have if they later developed breast cancer and had not availed themselves of screening.

The recent report of rising rates of contralateral prophylactic mastectomies—removing the unaffected breast in women with cancer in the other breast—in the United States indicates that the impact of this converged decision making is significant. The number of women diagnosed with cancer in one breast who had a prophylactic mastectomy in the unaffected breast rose from 1.8 percent in 1998 to 4.5 percent in 2003.[23] Although accurate statistics are not yet available, there is reason to believe that rates of prophylactic mastectomies for women "merely" at high risk for breast cancer, whether identified as such by genetic screening or on other grounds, have been climbing along with the rates for women with diagnosed breast cancer.[24] In other words, the converged experience is reflected in the parallel decision making of those people who are at risk for disease and those who have manifest yet very different stages of disease.

Neither improvements in surgery nor new biomedical insights are, in my view, by themselves driving such rapid change. It is revealing that the incidence of prophylactic surgery for women with breast cancer increased for women at every stage, at an almost identical slope.[25] Decision making about prophylactic surgery does not appear to have been based solely on straightforward calculations of altered probabilities of future cancer among women at different degrees of risk and disease. From a rational decision-making perspective, we would expect that women at a lower risk of recurrence would have a lower rate of change, since they have less to gain from this severely mutilating operation (their absolute rates are, in fact, lower). The fact that women of all stages share equally in the increasing rate of prophylactic surgery suggests that they are being exposed to some common external influence. Some observers have pinpointed the reasons for this increase, such as the use of more sensitive diagnostic and screening technologies (e.g., breast MRIs), which I am sure are operative.[26] But also important is the way that people at different points in the actively constructed risk continuum experience risk in similar ways and use similar decision-making strategies and styles, relatively autonomous from the objective probabilities of bad outcomes.

Although I would not want to second-guess any particular individual's decision, I find troubling the rapid and uniform rise in prophylactic surgery at all points in the risk continuum. Clinical or policy responses should take into account the active role of knowledge production about risk and risk-reducing practices in generating fear and overselling, in my estimation, the efficacy of current risk-reducing efforts. Blurring the boundary between risk and disease in decision making is facilitated by the way that we name and classify risk and disease. Many clinicians now recognize that a pathological diagnosis after breast biopsy of lobular carcinoma in situ (LCIS) is, in essence, the discovery of an underlying state of *risk* but that the cancer terminology, along with its embodied character, makes it much more frightening and encourages decision-making styles typically used in symptomatic and more advanced cancer. This semantic slippage and other negative aspects of the converged disease experience, such as the overselling of fear and fear-reducing interventions by the pharmaceutical industry and others, might be mitigated by more critical attention to the way we define, name, and classify cancer and other diseases.

The convergence of risk and disease has also led to a larger and more highly mobilized disease/risk population with expanded markets for interventions and greater clout for disease advocates. Combining people with prehypertension and frank hypertension and with prediabetes and diabetes, for example has enlarged the market for hypertension and diabetes medication. In addition, the enlarged size of the risk/disease population can lead to more visible and effective disease advocacy, which can then bring greater political pressure for funding basic and clinical research, which itself can contribute—via even more expanded definitions of risk and disease—to increases in the mobilized population. Again, this is most visible in the rapid growth in breast cancer advocacy in the United States over the past few decades, but similar trends can be seen in other risk/disease populations, such as the one formed by a convergence of obesity and type 2 diabetes. As these highly mobilized, converged risk/disease populations are often constituted by the marketing of tests and products, often by players with narrow economic interests (such as pharmaceutical companies, device manufacturers, and doctors influenced by them), we need a more vigorous and skeptical response to the active attempts to converge individuals at different points in the risk continuum into large markets for interventions and products.

The converged experience of risk and disease has also led to dramatic shifts in the perceived severity and spectrum of the disease, with ripple effects on how people experience and understand their illness. The expanded risk continuum makes people with a poor prognosis and rapidly advancing disease much more of a minority than in the past and makes the public face of some transformed diseases seem healthier and in general helps put a veneer of optimism onto the expanded group's identity. One of my students with long-standing type 1 diabetes has been upset by media reports that a famous actress, previously a spokesperson for the disease, had been able to wean herself off insulin. She suspected that the actress's original diagnosis was due to the blurring of type 1 diabetes, type 2 diabetes, and prediabetes.[27] My student worried that the glib media message of self-cure and control created impossible expectations for type 1 diabetic patients and undermined public appreciation of the serious challenges that type 1 diabetics face. In the many less far-fetched instances in which the experiences of highly symptomatic individuals are drowned out by the expanded risk/disease continuum, it might be appropriate to uphold or reinvent more categorical distinctions between risk and highly symptomatic disease.

One last consequence of the convergence of risk and disease is the proliferation of interventions promising both risk reduction and efficacy against symptomatic disease. Before data from the Women's Health Initiative appeared, many women were encouraged to take sex hormones both to control menopausal symptoms and to reduce the risk of chronic disease later in life. Menopause had been constructed partly as a symptomatic condition and partly as another "at risk" state. The bundling of risk reduction and disease treatment also is evident in the market niche of many new drugs whose sole or main selling point is the promise to put patients at less risk from particular side effects than competing drugs do. For example, the COX-2 inhibitor class of nonsteroidal anti-inflammatory drugs, like Vioxx and Celebrex, were promoted as being as efficacious as existing pain relievers and anti-inflammatory drugs but putting patients at less risk of gastrointestinal bleeding. Their remarkable market success followed from this combination of efficacy against disease and symptoms and promise to be less risky than competing drugs. But risk reduction is subject to an "easy come, easy go" principle, as elaborated in the next chapter. Knowledge of imposed risks can quickly undermine a drug's risk-reducing rationale. As quickly as the risk of COX-2 inhibitors dominated the anti-inflammatory market, so did this market share collapse with evidence that they increased cardiovascular risk. It is hard to promote the efficacy of a risk-modifying intervention as reducing fear and uncertainty when the very same intervention causes fear and uncertainty.

Combining risk reduction with symptomatic relief is a subspecies of the larger way that risk reduction has permeated not just disease prevention for the healthy but the experience and management of existing disease. Bundling risk reduction and symptom relief may be a good thing in itself, but in many instances, it is part of a problematic, self-reinforcing cycle of fear promotion followed by the marketing of tests and products that promise some means to reassert control over fear.

These cycles of risk production and risk reduction in our primary and secondary prevention efforts have financial and psychological costs. Should we have a higher bar for accepting new practices and products whose primary goal is to reduce the risk of other practices and products? As I discuss in chapter 5, recent arguments about the cost-effectiveness of new HPV vaccines show that the substantial savings might ensue not so much from the reduction of morbidity and mortality from cervical cancer and other HPV-related diseases but instead from reduced HPV-related Pap smear abnormalities and the expensive and intrusive workups they trigger. This is a real and important saving, but there is also something futile and problematic about this kind of meta-efficacy in which risk interventions reduce the costs and harms of other risk interventions, especially if such practices become dominant in our clinical and public health work.

Conclusions

I have emphasized the generally underappreciated and often unsettling consequences of the transformed chronic disease experience and its convergence with the experience of risk. We cannot set back the clock, nor would we want to. But we can do more to reduce the financial costs, disturbance to peace of mind, and distractions from other health goals that are the downsides of the converged experience.

Many of the changes that I have described are the result of one form or another of knowledge production, especially research into the natural history of disease and the construction of new risk states within existing chronic disease. Additional influences have been secondary or spillover effects of the ways in which we diagnose and treat chronic disease. Yet neither this knowledge production nor these late effects of existing clinical practices are typically understood as central issues in policy analysis or response.

Our current policies generally respond to different risk-reducing interventions—screening or diagnostic tests, preventative medications, and lifestyle changes—one at a time, in isolation from one another, and only after they have a foothold in clinical practice. Policy makers generally do not ask, for example, why some risks and not others are researched and promoted. We do not generally evaluate the cumulative effects of different prevention practices or the ways that new treatments and surveillance regimes expand and legitimate the risk states they target. We have also placed much less evidence-based scrutiny on the surveillance of existing disease and "secondary prevention" compared with primary prevention. Current cost-effectiveness analyses of, say, a new surveillance routine for someone who has had cancer, however evidence based, do not typically capture the cumulative effects on the peace of mind or the work of patienthood of many such practices. When existing definitions of disease are expanded, we do not generally measure consequences such as the increased fear that often follows from the higher prevalence and visibility of a condition.

The transformed disease experience suggests a different kind of evaluation and policy response from the present status quo, one that examines the "upstream" processes resulting in knowledge production about risks and new preventive practices and products (see chapter 9). Our policies need to evaluate and regulate the processes by which risks are named, identified, and researched; how the demand for intervention is produced; and what the many spillover effects of our risk interventions are.

We might, for example, expand the current regulatory oversight of direct-to-consumer advertising of prescription drugs to include weighing the impact of creating much larger markets composed of both the "at risk for" and the already diseased. We might insist that marketers maintain a stricter boundary between disease and risk in labeling and advertising. In funding research and formulating best clinical practices, we could respond more skeptically to research, product development, and calls for clinical and behavioral change that assume an unmitigated good from "early" intervention in disease. Such scrutiny already exists in oversight bodies like the U.S. Preventive Services Task Force when it evaluates claims for primary prevention (preventing disease from appearing in the first place). But there is much less awareness when evaluating "risk-reducing" interventions against existing disease.

It is, of course, difficult to measure consequences such as fear, disturbance to peace of mind, and the work of patienthood and to balance these effects against the health benefits of new knowledge and practices. But focusing only on what is easy to measure and value will not banish the challenges posed by the converged experience of risk and chronic disease.

3

The social and psychological efficacy of risk interventions

Will twenty-second century observers look back at American consumption of risk-reducing drugs and risk-reducing practices the way
we in the present look back at the bleeding and purging done in early
nineteenth-century America? They might wonder why there was so
much enthusiasm for many risk interventions for which there was
often no conclusive evidence that they improved health or saved lives.

Looked at another way, healers and patients two hundred years
ago were neither illogical nor irrational and neither are we today.
As Charles Rosenberg showed in his analysis of traditional American medical therapeutics, efficacy depends on shared assumptions
about how the body works and how health and illness are defined.
The efficacy of traditional therapeutic practices, such as bleeding or
the administration of purgatives and laxatives, was tightly connected
to the belief that these practices redressed the humoral and other imbalances that constituted ill health. Both doctor and patient required
evidence that treatments were efficacious in these terms. The very material and observable effects on the body that these treatments caused,
e.g., loss of blood, vomiting, and diarrhea, were witnessed and served
as evidence that humoral balance was being restored. In traditional
parlance, drugs were "exhibited," emphasizing the performative and
ritualized nature of therapeutics.[1]

Today the risk-reducing medicine's impact on the body is witnessed, albeit in a more virtual way, by such things as reduced serum
cholesterol levels and made meaningful by a body metaphor in which

health is the net vector of risk-producing and risk-lowering lifestyles, medicines, and practices.[2] In both traditional therapeutics and our present approaches, there is a system with similar constitutive elements: sense-giving assumptions about the body, health, and illness; a central role for witnessed evidence; and "props" that support the more ritualized and performative aspects of interventions. And these constitutive elements are adapted to their social and economic contexts: the home-based and often intimate doctor-patient relationship of the nineteenth century and the increasingly bureaucratic and third party–dominated present.

I stress these continuities with traditional medicine (which is of course a much more complicated and diverse set of ideas, technologies, and practices than my brief description conveys), despite the fact that modern therapeutics is unquestionably much more effective at saving lives and reducing morbidity as well as being based on superior scientific understanding and empirical evidence. These continuities provide an opportunity to rethink and reimagine present therapeutics in a more comprehensive way. They also can help make sense of our dilemmas over the costs and quality of health care today.

There is little scientific basis for the extensive geographic variation in patterns of medical practice. Some medical interventions persist long after they have been shown to be ineffective. Policy makers often deplore our inability to discipline wasteful or inefficient medical practices. But we have rarely asked why "ineffective" and often costly interventions exist in the first place. Why do some interventions diffuse rapidly in medical practice and patient/consumer behavior prior to or independent of the production of evidence of efficacy and safety? I believe that risk interventions often do a lot of *work* besides their actual or putative impact on objective health states. Understanding this other *work* can help explain these perplexing, often "evidence-free" patterns of diffusion.

It is also often assumed that more and improved scientific and clinical evidence and increased efforts at objective evaluation of such evidence are a sufficient response to our present cost and quality problems. The expanding universe of the highest-quality recommendations drawn from the best clinical trials and expert consensus conferences has been given the label *evidence-based medicine*. Like the "complete operation" for cancer in the early twentieth century, a.k.a. radical cancer surgery, which in one rhetorical stroke made any other surgery "incomplete," who today would own up to practicing, as a friend often quips, *evidence-free medicine*?[3] Yet there is a lot of evidence that there is inadequate evidence for many medical practices and products.[4] Why does this situation persist?

The typical answer is that there is not enough evidence, or the evidence is not adequately diffused to decision makers, or the evidence exists and is known but is resisted because economic and other incentives are aligned against otherwise best practices. These answers assume that what needs to be explained and corrected are the obstacles to physicians, patients, and consumers doing what is generally understood to be best practices as well as redressing knowledge gaps. Missing in this *deficit* approach is recognition that there exist alternative ways of deciding which practices and products work and what work they do. From this perspective, much of modern medical and health-consumer practice has not simply failed to use evidence, but is operating under a different set of assumptions and influences about what efficacy means and *is*.[5]

This chapter explores what we mean by efficacy, the power to have an effect, in the increasing number of health and health care decisions that have the goal of reducing risk—calls for behavioral change, screening programs, preventive drugs, etc. Their efficacy is necessarily understood in a different way than that of practices that directly and immediately impact symptoms from, or signs of, disease. Their efficacy often involves some leap of faith, trusting in results of epidemiological or clinical research rather than perceived effects on the body.

My approach draws from the important anthropological literature on the myriad ways people in different societies make sense of therapies, especially the extensive ethnographic literature on how different cultures construct the efficacy of medications.[6] "Consumers do not have the technological know-how to measure the pharmacological effects of a medicine," Whyte et al. convincingly argue. "This inability to measure efficacy leaves room for the most divergent ideas about medicines, varying from 'chemical poison' to 'miraculous power.'"[7] But the social and psychological efficacy of risk interventions in affluent countries does not exist solely because consumers lack the technical know-how to evaluate claims about pharmacological or any other type of more scientific efficacy. It also results from a system of beliefs and routines that includes biomedical knowledge and its production. This efficacy does not constitute an alternative or counterculture nor is it confined to the consumer realm.

When I evoke *scientific efficacy*, I am referring to the power to positively influence some measureable health parameter as established by rigorous clinical experimentation. Others have researched the history of modern clinical experimentation and its impact on medical practice and thought.[8] My focus is the actions and decisions of individual consumers, patients, and health care workers. Efficacy as established in clinical trials is relevant to these actors, but often indirectly, more the way a *Consumer Reports* evaluation of toasters is relevant to the individual consumer. He or she may have read such a report and found it useful, but the decision to buy or not may be swayed by factors that were not or could not be rigorously evaluated. Given the low price and ease with which a toaster can be replaced, objective and quantitative evidence of durability might not be relevant to the would-be purchaser. Instead, the most relevant parameter might be the product's stainless steel look.

So below I offer two sets of reflections. The first is an overview of the social and psychological work done by modern risk interventions. The second covers the ways—besides the strength of medical evidence—that doctors, patients, and consumers in recent decades have been persuaded that risk interventions are efficacious.[9] Many risk interventions diffuse before their scientific efficacy has been established or even tested by rigorous clinical experiments. Understanding how and why this happens is crucial to formulating workable responses to many current dilemmas in disease prevention practices and policies.

The social and psychological efficacy of modern risk interventions

In addition to whatever impact risk interventions have on the probabilities of suffering disease and ill health, they also provide a means to control the uncertainty and fear associated with disease. This is especially true for cancer, which is greatly feared not only because of the disease's destructiveness and lethality, but also because cancer awareness programs and early detection and diagnosis have led many people to believe that they are at increased risk of contracting it.[10]

It is not surprising then that many women under fifty with no family history of breast cancer get screening mammograms, and some doctors advocate them, despite evidence that they are either ineffective at saving lives or have some minimal impact but incur substantial physical and financial costs. Many women and their doctors feel that a screening mammogram is the only positive action they can take to allay their fears and control the uncertainty associated with being at risk for cancer. At the same time, screening mammography has played a large role in creating these fears and uncertainties. The frightening 1:8 lifetime odds of developing breast cancer that American women face is a direct consequence of the massive increase in cancer diagnoses that followed the introduction and uptake of mass screening. The resulting self-reinforcing cycle of risk creation and risk reduction helps explain the high penetration and durability of screening mammography even in populations for which there is minimal evidence of scientific efficacy.

The experience of being at risk for disease is not only a psychological response to the probabilities of this or that outcome. It is also constituted by predictable and structured routines, resulting in a characteristic risk experience or state. This *risk state* may be similar to the experience of bona fide disease. Risk is also often embodied, adding to its disease-ness.[11] Some risk interventions are aimed at preventing this risk state as much as or more than the targeted condition.

One striking example of this risk state is the life of a woman who tests positive for human papilloma virus (HPV) infection. Because persistent HPV infection is known to be a cause of cervical and other cancers, women who test positive become part of a class of people who often have repeated cytological tests for cancer (Pap smears and HPV DNA probes) and undergo interventions such as cryotherapy (freezing parts of the cervix identified as abnormal).[12] They may also experience the stigma of carrying a sexually transmitted disease (STD) that can lead to cancer not only for oneself but for sexual partners. And this sexual transmission is not easily prevented by condoms or other means.

Avoiding this state of risk—including the costs and uncertainties of repeated testing and interventions—is a major efficacy of the new HPV vaccines. While the risk-reducing nature of these vaccines is explored in detail in chapter 5, I want to underscore here that these vaccines, in common with other risk interventions, often promise some relief from the risk state itself as much or more than the targeted biomedical condition.[13] This point is well illustrated by a Merck informational website devoted to HPV that features four "real life" video stories. "That's right, real. We wanted to hear from the people who are getting vaccinated—in their own words. We also wanted to hear from people whose lives have already been affected by human papillomavirus (HPV). Take a look, then talk to your doctor or health care professional."[14]

In one of the video stories, a young, articulate middle-class woman sits in the front seat of a car. The jerky video and unbalanced framing create the impression that she is being filmed by a friend next to her, more homemade video than the slick corporate product that it is. Her voice trembling, she tells us that she has been infected with HPV for over six years. She says things are OK but exudes fear and worry. "It's important to know the state of your body," she advises. "As women, our bodies are so fragile and we need to take care of them. And we need to know what's going on. So I get checkups every six months. I get Pap smears. And every six months they come back that I have HPV. But it's OK. Because I am healthy. I don't have any signs of cancer or precancer." The video concludes with the narrator imploring other women to get checkups and "know your status at all times."

The not-so-subtle message in this real-life story is that being HPV positive, an embodied *state of risk* for cervical cancer, is something to be avoided at all costs. While she states "I am healthy," presumably meaning she does not have cervical cancer, being positive for HPV on repeated Pap smears is shown to be a serious condition in itself, constituted by feeling contaminated and contagious. Gardasil, Merck's vaccine, is never mentioned but the message from this story and the other ones on this website is clear. Take the vaccine and avoid ending up like this woman—wracked with fear, uncertainty, and regret and living a life filled with frequent tests and the potentially fateful consequences of their results. In other words, the vaccine's efficacy is not so much against *cervical cancer*, which is, after all, rare, often preventable by interventions triggered by abnormal Pap smears, and much more likely to impact poor and marginalized women, but this frightening *state of risk*. This efficacy is real, important for all women (not just woman at special risk of cancer), and immediate. Another apparently middle-class woman whose real life story appears on this site tells us that she "felt a huge sense of relief" as soon as she was vaccinated.

This "risk-reducing" social or psychological efficacy has not been studied or proven in a clinical trial. In informational sites, direct-to-consumer advertisements, and physician detailing, this efficacy may be central to decision making but only hinted at, as in this "real life" story pitch. It is left up to the consumer or patient to fill in the blanks. This indirectness follows partly from regulatory constraints that limit claims not based on scientific evidence. But appeals to fear and convenience may also be more persuasive if left inexplicit.

As with being HPV positive, other risk states can be worrisome, consequential, and involve work, and so be something to avoid. This is especially true of many embodied cancer risk states such as having "abnormal cells of uncertain significance" on a Pap test, a high PSA level on a screening test, or a breast biopsy showing lobular carcinoma in situ (LCIS). These risks also often lead to more surveillance, problematic decisions, and a strong desire to push the reset button to an earlier time when the risks were unknown.

The risk state is not something confined to cancer and cancer screening. For years I worked in a travel medicine clinic. Patients/consumers wanted vaccinations and preventive medications, each of which had its indications and contraindications. The underlying motivation for coming to the clinic, however, was often to take precautionary steps so that the travel experience would be pleasurable rather than dominated by a heightened sense of disease risk. As I show in chapter 6, Lyme disease vaccination was (unsuccessfully) sold to residents of high-risk areas as a way to change their fear and risk-inflected relationship with their local environment.[15]

Given that risk states are often experienced as chronic, ever-present conditions, it is not surprising that some *continuous* interventions have diffused widely in medical practice without evidence of their superior scientific efficacy over intermittent interventions and sometimes in the face of efforts to reduce their use. Perhaps the most striking example of the appeal of this social and psychological efficacy is the decades-long use of continuous fetal heart monitoring for rou-

tine maternal labor. Scientific evidence has accumulated either showing no benefit or limited benefit (small reduction in neonatal seizures)
over one or two evaluations of fetal heart rate by stethoscope and at
the cost of increased frequency of caesarian sections and invasive
vaginal deliveries.[16] Yet hospitals routinely use the technology. In part,
continuous fetal monitoring diffused before there was any scientific
evidence at all. Once part of everyday practice, it has been especially
difficult for obstetricians and mothers to wean themselves from the
seemingly objective means of monitoring changes in the fetus' status.
Over the past century, obstetricians and others have transformed
labor into a highly intervened-in risk state. The constant surveillance
provided by these monitors gives immediate and continuous reassurance to both doctor and patient. Of course, such reassurance persists
until abnormalities develop, many of which are borderline and difficult to interpret.[17]

In the very different setting of pharmaceutical cancer preventatives, a similar logic often holds. Some women with breast cancer who
take the antiestrogen Tamoxifen for the recommended five years have
been reluctant to stop despite the lack of evidence (until very recently)
that there is net benefit after this period is over.[18] Breast cancer risk
feels continuous and persists after initial treatment, so there may be
something reassuring about uninterrupted, continuous preventative
interventions. This kind of efficacy also helps explain why controversy
erupts whenever recommendations are made to lengthen the intervals between this or that cancer screening test.

Similar social and psychological efficacy considerations may help
explain the quick and relatively evidence-free diffusion of routine
ultrasonography in obstetrical practice. Ultrasounds are done routinely in pregnancy. They provide both doctor and patient with reassurance against the continuous risks and concerns associated with
pregnancy. It took active resistance and our physician clout for my
psychiatrist wife and me to ward off the many attempts to do routine
ultrasounds during my wife's pregnancy with our second child a few
decades ago. We preferred not learning about some abnormality we
could not remedy or a false positive finding over the small chance of
learning about some risk that we might act upon.

In addition to interventions whose social and psychological efficacy is to reduce risk of disease or health problems, the efficacy of

many medications and interventions is often that they are less risky than other practices or interventions. The market niche of one class of analgesics (which also have anti-inflammatory effects), the COX-2 inhibitors (Vioxx, Celebrex), was that they had less risk of gastrointestinal side effects than existing nonsteroidal anti-inflammatory medications. Ironically, but not unexpectedly, these mass-marketed medications ended up themselves connected with increased health risks, as COX-2 inhibitors were associated with cardiovascular disease and ignited controversy, lawsuits, and practice change.

How have we been persuaded to believe that risk interventions work? What sustains their use?

That many risk-reducing interventions alleviate or eliminate states of fear, uncertainty, and lack of control—whether or not there is evidence of scientific efficacy—does not by itself explain their often rapid and widespread diffusion. It is only a commonplace to say to oneself "I am feeling pretty healthy . . . got checked out by my doctor and my cholesterol, blood pressure, and cancer screening tests are all within normal limits. I exercise regularly and avoid unhealthy foods, etc." But how have we been persuaded that normal values of risk factors and compliance with behavioral norms are credible evidence of health (or in many cases, constitutes health)? Or, if abnormal, are worth triggering further tests and interventions? We do not typically feel better or suffer any symptom less after taking a lipid or blood pressure–lowering pill or experiencing a cancer screening test. Evidence of scientific efficacy may exist, but that evidence often bears little in the way of dose-response relationship to the uptake of interventions. Moreover, the acceptance of the efficacy of risk interventions is a sociohistorical process as well as an individual one, often based on developments that have occurred long before any individual physician or patient/consumer takes a pill or changes his or her behavior.

The acceptance of the efficacy of a risk-reducing intervention often involves a leap of faith. People who take risk-reducing medicines typically experience no relief from symptoms but often have side effects. They persevere because they trust that the probability of some bad outcome has been reduced. Consider those people who take drugs that promise to modify the course of Alzheimer's disease, mentioned in the previous chapter. People on these medicines still have progressive disease and typically get worse over time. Family members and physicians are often persuaded to use these medicines trusting in the counterfactual, that the affected individual would have been even worse without the medication.[19]

One historical precondition for being persuaded that many twentieth- and twenty-first-century risk interventions are effective was the earlier broad shift in the medical model of ill health. In the nineteenth century, as humoral views of the body waned and ill health was increasingly understood in terms of specific mechanistically defined disease, both traditional therapeutics and a way of thinking about efficacy and evidence were undermined. Efficacy was no longer restoration of individual humoral balance, but increasingly became the power to have an effect on the natural history of a specific disease. Interventions that changed symptoms and signs or laboratory values believed to be associated with different steps in a disease's natural history were increasingly understood as efficacious. Because we understand that exposure to specific risks over time and in predictable ways leads to disease, we are ready to accept changes in risk markers as evidence of efficacy.

The dense web of knowledge about the natural history of disease has become the scaffolding upon which many risk interventions are built. The denser the knowledge of predisposing factors and disease stages, and the more they are accepted within a natural history narrative, the more opportunities there are for intervention. When strokes and heart attacks and Alzheimer's disease were understood as chronic degenerative diseases, resulting from nonspecific wear and tear and aging, there were few calls to disease prevention of any sort.[20]

Interventions have at the same time stabilized our beliefs about and models of the natural history of disease. Interventions have sometimes reinforced the legitimacy and naturalness of the risk stratification, transforming the way we understand the natural history of disease. So, for example, analysis of clinical trial data revealed that men and women with either three occluded coronary vessels or disease of the left main artery benefited from bypass surgery while people with "lesser" or different types of coronary obstruction did as well on medical therapy. This risk stratification was then used in both clinical trials and routine practice and influenced the way cardiologists and others think and talk about the natural history of disease. We now typically talk about "three-vessel disease" as a natural category to be treated with a specific intervention. A similar process has occurred with "estrogen receptor positive" breast cancer, where a well-accepted type of cancer is now defined by its response to (anti)estrogen treatment.

Clinical experiments as scientific endorsements

The scientific plausibility of many disease risks and the efficacy of many risk interventions were established by large-scale epidemiological studies and clinical trials at midcentury. For example, the Framingham Heart Study, explored in the next chapter, was the seminal cohort study of risk factors for coronary heart disease. It was launched in 1948 and produced knowledge about risk factors that soon became the targets of major interventions—drugs to control hypertension and hyperlipidemia, but also major diet, exercise, and other initiatives.

Since at least the 1950s, the "gold standard" for establishing efficacy of these and other interventions has been the randomized clinical trial (RCT). Although the epitome of scientific methods for establishing the efficacy of medical interventions, RCT results are almost never unambiguous. There are also contested extrapolations to real-world conditions and different populations than those studied. Trial results also need to be considered in the context of other data and practices. The particular nature of many risk interventions—often aimed at large populations who until they were screened or clinically tested were unaware that they had a problem—suggests that there should be a very high bar for good evidence of efficacy before interventions are diffused.

Clinical experiments have played a central role in persuading clinicians and others that particular interventions work, but evidence per se is not the only aspect of clinical experiments that is persuasive. Clinical trials have also been persuasive in less transparent and objective ways. In marketing, displays of evidence from clinical trials can function as a kind of seal of endorsement from science, over and above the purely cognitive and logical implications of evidence.[21] This is apparent from the rapid increase in direct-to-consumer advertising (DTCA) of prescription medicines, legalized in 1998 and now a major part of the medical marketplace, but also in physician-targeted print advertisements in earlier eras. The claims made by these advertisements are regulated, but given the constraints of a sixty-second commercial or journal page, no real communication of the strengths and weaknesses of scientific results is possible or expected.[22] Yet claims made in such advertisements are supposed to be backed up by clinical trial data and often there are explicit citations of trials in advertisements.

Highly stylized presentations of the results of clinical and other experiments have long been used in advertisements for consumer goods, especially ones with a health rationale, like toothpaste or cleansing agents. Health-promoting products have long been central to American marketing, from the medicine show and patent medicines in the nineteenth century to the DTCA of drugs today.[23] Many of these products have considerable social and psychological efficacy, i.e., they satisfy the consumer need for reassurance, relief from worry, proof of being a good mother, etc.

Claims made about future objective health benefits were part and parcel of selling products like Listerine since the early decades of the twentieth century. Listerine freshened the mouth, an effect that could be linked to everything from attracting a mate to success in business. At the same time, advertisers linked Listerine to health gains like fewer colds and less severe infections. Advertisements for Listerine were full of quantitative claims of germ reduction and also evidence from unreferenced clinical trials showing other health impacts.[24]

Along similar lines, by the 1950s marketers deployed the emerging gold standard for scientific efficacy—the blind randomized controlled trial—to persuade consumers to buy health-related consumer products. The efficacy of Crest toothpaste, for example, rested on claims that the fluoride it contained reduced cavities. In a series of television commercials, viewers were exposed to a series of randomized trials of schoolchildren and students at a military boarding school who were assigned to toothpaste A or B (one of which was Crest) and followed to see cavity rates. Later, investigators identified which group received Crest; this group had much lower cavity rates. These demonstrations were accompanied by more traditional consumer pitches to less scientific endpoints, such as proving one is a good parent (i.e., the repeated scene of an excited child running into his mother's arms with news from the dentist: "look ma, no cavities"). There were also testimonies of better mouth taste and the rewards that followed from better breath—greater sex appeal and success in school, work, and dating—echoing earlier Listerine claims.[25]

Were consumers swayed by this demonstration? And if they were, was it because the television endorsement led to a calculation that the evidence of benefit was worth any putative costs? Perhaps, but the product—with its multiple purposes and uses—was also more attractive because of the scientific aura attached to the exhibition of results from clinical trials, in a manner that resembles the persuasive power of a celebrity endorsement more than the objective assessment of evidence. Such exhibitions and endorsements associate the product with something or someone positive. Consumer and advertiser engage in a joint fantasy that the product exhibited is attractive and worth buying. Like claims that nine out of ten doctors prefer to smoke a particular cigarette, which were once common in cigarette advertising, the clinical trial established a connection between the product and a previously established good thing (medicine, doctors).[26]

It is hard to say what present-day consumers make of claims of efficacy from clinical trial data that appear in DTCA, or in newspaper stories, or from their doctors. My hunch is that "clinical trials" and other knowledge-making practices have been persuasive in ways similar to these Crest advertisements. These practices persuade at multiple interacting levels. As a result, the boundaries between scientific efficacy, on the one hand, and different social and psychological efficacies, on the other, are, often purposely, blurred. This system of persuasion operates whether the scientific rationale for the intervention is robust or weak, although it is much more apparent when evidence is weak or the object of persuasion is a consumer product that is not claimed to have a significant impact on morbidity or mortality.

Autocatalytic cycles of risk production and reduction

Risk-reducing practices can create their own demand. In this way, the efficacy of some risk interventions is *reflexive*. Reflexivity is sometimes used by social scientists to denote situations in which actors observing or theorizing about some social system unknowingly impact it. Observations and theories that are meant to be objective accounts of some phenomenon are in fact contributing to it.[27] Risk interventions can be reflexive when belief in their efficacy drives their uptake, creating conditions that further cement belief in their efficacy, leading to more uptake, etc. Reflexivity captures an important way in which doctors, patients, and consumers have been persuaded that risk interventions are effective.

Reflexivity is not new to historians of disease.[28] Ludwik Fleck, in the 1930s, made an analogy between the medical researcher or physician and his perceptions of disease to the situation of a "casual visitor to the Stock Exchange, who feels the panic selling in a bear market as only an external force existing in reality. He is completely unaware of his own excitement in the throng and hence does not realize how much he may be contributing to the general state." Fleck made this analogy as part of a general epistemological argument that we understand scientific thinking and practice, especially regarding disease and its causes, as socially constructed, collective processes.[29]

George Soros, hedge fund manager and philanthropist, has in a different domain argued that there is a reflexive relationship between economic actors and the market fundamentals they are theoretically observing. He used the example of oil prices to make this point. Rising oil prices should motivate increased production but instead can be understood as a reason to keep oil in the ground. With prices rising, oil will be or is perceived to be worth more in the future. With further restriction in supply due to such beliefs, oil prices continue to rise: a self-perpetuating system that goes on until the bubble bursts. In the boom phase of bubbles, many participants are aware that prices are rising to unsupportable levels by a kind of groupthink that is divorced from economic fundamentals, but actors at the same time may feel, especially in a competitive situation, that they have to "dance until the music stops playing," i.e., they will lose out, at least in the short run relative to others, if they do not participate in these cycles.

In a similar way, our ideas about disease fundamentals (such as the causes of morbidity and mortality) can influence rather than simply reflect those fundamentals. In the case of risk interventions, observers assess whether, say, a screening test triggers actions that reduce the chances of getting a disease and suffering the most feared consequences. But observers do not passively observe some objective change in these consequences. Their beliefs and perceptions—and the actions they take in response—shape how efficacy is constructed.

A central example of reflexivity in risk interventions is the relationship among disease prevention efforts, perceptions of efficacy, and changed routines. Many early to mid-twentieth century cancer prevention efforts aimed to get women to medical care as soon as they recognized of one of six cancer danger signs. This "do not delay" campaign impacted individual and physician behavior. Reflexivity manifested itself. As more and more individuals complied with this campaign, the case fatality rate—of the people with the disease, the proportion that die—got smaller. This apparent sign of progress occurs when many more people are diagnosed without much or any change in the numbers of people dying from the disease. The falling case fatality is an entirely predictable result of diagnosing more people with cancer yet having no change in the numbers who die, as was the case for many cancers during this period. This improved case fatality was widely attributed to the efficacy of then current clinical and public health actions, and led to greater compliance with the early detection message, leading to further apparent improvement in case fatality (and its inverse, the survival rate). The greater numbers of cancer diagnoses without significant impact on mortality might have curtailed our screening paradigm but—like the processes that keep high-priced oil in the ground—instead led to a perception that cancer survival has increased, which along with increased fear, led to more screening, and so on.[30]

Recruits increase, disease definition broadens, and efficacy increases

For some people the absence of disease or disease progression is persuasive evidence for the efficacy of risk interventions. A joke from my childhood depends on similar epistemological chicanery. "Why do elephants wear green pajamas?" I would ask. "I don't know" the stumped listener would reply. "In order to camouflage themselves on pool tables. Ever see an elephant on a pool table?" "No," says the listener. "You see, it works."

Many disease states targeted by risk interventions are assumed to be progressive and prevalent. So when the target disease does not develop in a person at high risk or diagnosed with "early" disease after a risk intervention, many people assume, following the green pajamas logic, that the intervention worked. For example, one of the most powerful reasons why prostate cancer screening is widely endorsed is

the existence of a large and ever-increasing number of apparent prostate cancer survivors. This growing number is assumed to be a sign
of success, when another interpretation is that many more people
are being diagnosed and treated who would have otherwise died of
other causes or could be successfully treated later if cancer developed.
Not developing the disease that one is putatively preventing, like the
invisibility of the elephant in green pajamas, is often persuasive evidence of the efficacy of risk interventions.

Witnessed evidence of risk reduction

Like the early nineteenth-century patient, the early twenty-first-
century patient seeks evidence that risk interventions are efficacious.
Rather than believing in the physical evidence of sweating and diarrhea, the twenty-first-century patient seeks other types of evidence,
usually evidence of biological impact from laboratory tests.

For example, the asymptomatic early twenty-first-century man
recruited into the diagnosis of prediabetes by screening tests needs
some evidence of the efficacy of the medicine given to treat the condition, usually an oral hypoglycemic agent that his doctor is urging him
to take. Unlike the typical nineteenth-century patient, he has no felt
symptoms to be relieved. Evidence exists, however. The twenty-first-
century prediabetic will learn that the medication is likely to lower his
serum blood glucose level. This change might be linked to some statistical advantage in evading the end-organ damage of diabetes, perhaps
expressed as reduced relative risk. The reduced blood glucose might
lead to "losing" a prior diagnosis of metabolic syndrome, since this
entity is defined by elevation of a set of metabolic risk factors that includes serum glucose. This witnessed evidence of effect may restore a
sense of well-being, banish fear, and allow a greater sense of control
over feelings of randomness.[31]

A consumer of statins similarly finds evidence of an effect in a
lowered serum cholesterol level. Statins—like the risk factor they
target—do not generally cause symptoms. This is not understood as
evidence of no effect, but rather that they are palatable and safe. The
doctor's ability to measure serum cholesterol as well as other serum
levels that are associated with potential dangers (some of which, like
liver function abnormalities, are part and parcel of the putative inter-

ference in the liver's metabolic functioning that is the rationale for the drug's use), serve as witnessed evidence of effect. The use of drugs and quantitative measurements of risk reduction also make the underlying risk target more disease-like. This social and psychological work is so important that it is hard to imagine *not measuring* serum lipids, even if there were good scientific evidence that such determinations were useless and unnecessary.[32]

When I first wrote the last sentence, I had in mind a thought experiment in which American physicians and patients were forced to give up routine serum cholesterol monitoring for people being treated with cholesterol lowering medications. Soon after, in 2013, a controversy erupted when the American College of Cardiology and American Heart Association actually issued new guidelines for managing cardiovascular risk which in fact jettisoned 2 key elements of the social and psychological efficacy of risk management: (1) routine use of an individual's own high level of cholesterol as the primary threshold for intervention and (2) monitoring the efficacy of lipid lowering drugs with "evidence" of lowered serum cholesterol levels. Predictably, a firestorm of criticism and angst followed. The *New York Times* gave the controversy front page coverage and followed the story for weeks afterwards. In one article, my Penn colleague Dr. Dan Rader was quoted as saying that he "and other experts also worry that without the goal of target numbers, patients and their doctors will lose motivation to control cholesterol levels. 'They are used to it and believe in it.'" The same article cited prominent medical historian and internist Barron Lerner, who "gives patients a printout with their LDL levels circled before and after they started taking statins. "It is really helpful to have some kind of results to show people," says Lerner, adding, "I will predict 100% that I will have some patients who [will] say, 'If you are not going to check the LDL level and you cannot tell me the statin is working, then I am not going to take it.'"[33]

Giving a rational veneer for radical prevention

There may be less individualistic and more functional/structural reasons why some risk interventions have found their place in American medical practice without or in opposition to evidence of their scientific efficacy. Some risk interventions—especially cancer screening and risk stratification—persuade by legitimating and giving a rational veneer to extreme disease treatments that would otherwise be more difficult to justify and use.

So, for example, there is much controversy over whether routine PSA screening for prostate cancer testing is good policy. One of the most powerful arguments for its efficacy is the declining age-specific mortality from prostate cancer in the U.S. in the years after PSA screening was introduced. It is unclear how much of this decline is due to screening or other factors, such as improved treatment, or whether it represents a return to an earlier mortality baseline after years of increased screening-induced attention to the disease. Also, this decline could be at the expense of morbidity and mortality from complications due to prostate cancer interventions.

But there is one commonsense reason to find it plausible that screening leads to some decline in prostate cancer mortality. Screening leads to more biopsies and prostatectomies. Removing the prostate gland almost certainly results in some people being saved a prostate cancer death. This is true whether or not or the degree to which PSA correctly identifies people with cancer or being at high risk for deadly cancer. Prophylactic mastectomy, thyroidectomy, oophorectomy, and colectomy would likely have a similar effect on mortality from breast, thyroid, ovarian, and colon cancer.

Looked at this way, cancer screening tests can serve as a veneer for an extreme kind of prophylactic organ removal that would otherwise not be done to people at no special risk of disease. It is common today to represent the clinical utility of an intervention using the "numbers needed to screen/treat" metric (NNT). The "numbers needed to screen/treat to save one life" for some common cancer screening can be quite large and difficult to interpret and use for decision making. Some large but real NNT to save one life from a deadly cancer can exist without a test having much or any discriminative value. In other words the screening-biopsy-diagnosis-surgery-lowered mortality sequence of events is entirely predictable and independent of the screening test's actual net benefit.

Cancer screening would be experienced and understood very differently if the benefit for the test was in no small measure due to the number of organectomies the test induced in a population. We might be hard pressed to consent to screening tests if we understood them as roulette wheels, permitting a fraction of the population to get organs removed, some of which might be destined to later produce cancer. Yet we are persuaded of their efficacy by appeals that partly rest on this reality.

Why social and psychological efficacy matters

Myopic and flawed risk interventions are more likely to be developed and used when policy makers and clinicians do not take into account the social and psychological work they do. As I will describe in chapter 6, the market failure of the Lyme disease vaccines that appeared in the 1990s partly resulted from not understanding their specific social and psychological efficacy for particular groups and how easy it is to undermine a practice whose use is based on appeals to fear. The vaccine manufacturers did not fully appreciate that Lyme disease lay advocacy was focused on the legitimacy of chronic Lyme disease rather than fear of Lyme disease per se. For various reasons, the efficacy of the vaccine appeared to threaten the legitimacy of chronic Lyme disease. An alternative construction of vaccine efficacy, one in which the vaccine *caused* a Lyme disease–like syndrome via immune mechanisms, was understood to bolster the legitimacy of chronic Lyme disease. Disease advocates were able to undermine the vaccines market viability by publicizing these putative immune dangers. The failure of these vaccines illustrates a more general phenomenon—an intervention with plausible scientific efficacy but whose market viability depends on selling reassurance and reducing fear can be easily undermined by promoting the idea that the intervention itself poses risks, however small and theoretical. The life cycle of many modern risk interventions is often short, which I have characterized as following an "easy come, easy go" cycle.

There is of course the potential to use the social and psychological efficacy for good effect. I have semiseriously mused to medical colleagues that we might use the social and psychological efficacy of acupuncture to reduce antibiotic overuse and the resulting problems such as antibiotic resistance and adverse reactions. Efforts to educate prescribers that there is little net benefit to prescribing antibiotics for uncomplicated middle ear infections have been unsuccessful. Why not promote acupuncture, regardless of the lack of evidence of reduced pain or shorter duration of symptoms? Acupuncture might satisfy the need to do or prescribe something after a parent or adult has made the effort to seek medical attention for a painful condition while at the same time not contributing to the antibiotic overuse problem.

The social and psychological work done by many risk interventions can also help explain the mass expansion of risk interventions in the past few decades and why some persist and grow despite limited or no evidence of their efficacy. This expansion has been consequential. While not a zero-sum game, the expansion of risk interventions has taken away resources and attention we give to other types of interventions—to population-level prevention or the treatment of symptomatic progressive disease. The expansion of risk interventions, for example prostate cancer screening using prostate specific antigen levels, has led to inefficient use of resources, iatrogenic harm, and unending controversy.

"Being at risk for X . . ." is often a much more fungible and uniform state than suffering from a symptomatic disease. As a result, risks themselves and interventions to modify them can be readily expanded and also influenced by governments, large bureaucracies, and self-interested groups such as drug manufacturers and clinical specialists who stand to get more business. Interventions are also easily rationalized by appealing prevention rhetoric.

Moreover, risk interventions that have been approved for use after rigorous clinical trials are then sold to consumers, patients, and health professions by appeals to their social and psychological efficacy in medical detailing and DTCA (as in the HPV vignette discussed earlier). Few acknowledge this contradiction and "double dipping." On the one hand, interventions have the market protections and legitimacy of effective medical interventions proven or believed to be efficacious scientifically—long-duration and protected patent rights, access to insurance subsidies, and government support for prior research. On the other hand, they can be marketed and rationalized as consumer products.

At the same time, the patient or consumer contemplating whether to avail him or herself of a risk-reducing intervention—which characteristically produces no noticeable effect in itself—is typically in no position to judge from their own bodily or other individual experience whether it is actually effective or harmful. So he or she must rely on the promise of scientific knowledge production and regulatory protection. In this sense, the modern patient and consumer considering one or another risk intervention, although undoubtedly benefitting overall from the many scientific medical advances of the last century, is at the same time more vulnerable to manipulation and control from influences and processes that can be largely hidden from view. This vulnerability and potential for harm is the most compelling reason for a more informed skepticism about the expansion of risk states and interventions.

II

4

The Framingham Heart Study:
The emergence of the risk factor approach

Framingham and risk factors: "Out of this mountain of data . . ."

Beliefs about the causes of, and practices to prevent, coronary heart disease (CHD) changed dramatically in the decades after World War II. In the 1940s, most physicians and laypersons believed that angina pectoris and the other diseases and syndromes now subsumed under the CHD label represented a class of poorly understood degenerative heart diseases for which there was no effective prevention or treatment.

By the mid-1960s, however, medical and laypersons no longer believed that CHD was degenerative, random, and not preventable. Instead, they came to believe that CHD resulted from the interaction of multiple "risk factors," many of which could be modified by individual behavioral change or medical intervention. The new risk factor knowledge not only served as a scientifically based guide to individual behavior and to clinical and public health interventions, but as a framework for negotiating responsibility for CHD and for establishing social norms for what constitutes a healthy, good life.

In addition to the important advances in biomedical knowledge, what was also novel about the risk factor approach to CHD was a new *style* of explaining cause and responsibility, one that used probabilistic language to link quantifiable and elementary properties of individual physiology, behavior, and social and familial background to specific untoward outcomes. By the late 1960s, this style of explanation became the dominant way of expressing and conceptualizing what individuals contribute to CHD. How can we explain the emergence of the risk factor approach? Insofar as biomedical and lay people consider the remarkable changes in our beliefs about, and practices surrounding, CHD etiology and prevention, they most frequently assert that new, convincing, and scientifically valid data from epidemiologic research, most notably the Framingham Heart Study (which I will simply call Framingham), uncovered important etiologic associations that diffused through scientific and lay communities, radically changing the view of the disease as well as clinical and public health practices.

A writer for the *Boston Globe* in 1971 offered the following generally accepted view of the connection between Framingham and risk factors:

> Since 1949, 5127 citizens from the Boston suburb of 60,000 have reported faithfully every two years for physical exams which are conducted at a rate of 60 a week. Out of this mountain of data have come revelations on heart attack risk factors that have helped American physicians to devise preventive measures for high-risk patients. These risk factors—high blood pressure, cigarettes smoking, obesity, high blood-cholesterol levels and others—were either unknown or only guessed at prior to the Framingham study.[1]

The connection between Framingham and the emergence of the risk factor approach, however, is less a matter of cause and effect than such casual observations suggest. Prior to Framingham, the substantive knowledge about CHD predisposition that many people evoke with the term "risk factor" was not so much "unknown or only guessed at" as understood in a different way and put to different purposes. While Framingham helped usher in this new style and these new purposes, it was only one of many largely *social* influences on the emerging risk factor approach.

The structure, function, and significance of Framingham was itself in constant transition in the first twenty years of its existence, shaped at every point by social influences similar to those that led to the risk factor approach. Moreover, the appearance, structure, and scale of many other epidemiologic studies of CHD besides Framingham that appeared in the same short time period also reflect the importance of social influences on the emergence of the new risk factor consciousness in the 1950s and 1960s.[2]

By focusing on the changing identity of Framingham and its relationship to the emerging risk factor approach, I will contribute partial answers, subject to the limitations of a single historical case study, to two general lines of inquiry about the development of twentieth-century American medicine. First, how have novel research (in this case, epidemiological) methods and goals developed?[3] Framingham is a good case study for answering this question because of its frequent citation as the first comprehensive cohort study of the etiology of chronic disease and its long and well-documented history. Second, how and why have ideas about disease etiology and predisposition changed? Framingham's chronology roughly coincides with the emergence of the risk factor approach, and, as I already mentioned, many observers simply equate the two as cause and effect. By studying the internal history of Framingham and trying to build plausible connections between changes in the study's organization, hypotheses, goals, research reports, funding, and reception, on the one hand, and changing ideas about risk, responsibility, and cause of CHD, on the other, we can more precisely understand these interacting influences and the resulting changes in scientific and lay beliefs and practices.

I am indebted to a few observations made by Mervyn Susser about Framingham's role in the evolution of epidemiologic methods. Although Susser "discovered no true and complete precursor in epidemiology of the Framingham Study," he observed that what was novel about the study's methodology was not consciously planned by anyone but the result of a number of factors, especially the "requirements of studies of chronic disease."[4] His argument, like my own, follows from the observation that Framingham's novel features evolved in the course of the study.

I have divided Framingham's history into two phases: (1) epidemiologic approaches to CHD prior to Framingham through the study's early years (through 1951) and (2) the study's maturation (1952–70). By 1970, not only was Framingham an established and well-known study and its principal findings diffused to different audiences, but many contemporary risk factor beliefs and practices were established.

From "not preventable at the present time" to "the follow up study of normal persons": The origins of Framingham

Prevention of CHD in the 1930s and 1940s was most frequently discussed as "heart disease control" and was modeled on the much greater efforts at tuberculosis control. To control tuberculosis during this period, the U.S. Public Health Service (USPHS), for example, helped volunteer groups organize mass screening campaigns in communities and among special populations such as labor union members. After World War II, the USPHS encouraged general hospitals to routinely get chest X-rays on admitted patients. People who were identified as having tuberculosis might be sent to sanatoria for isolation and recuperation. These key elements of tuberculosis control—mass screening, early identification, reliance on voluntary efforts and community groups—were adopted throughout the Unites States.[5] The town of Framingham had itself been the site of a large "community health and tuberculosis demonstration" project in 1917 and 1918 that embodied these key elements.[6]

Analogous to this model, heart disease control generally meant the identification of cases with early disease, although there was little consensus about how to go about it. USPHS cardiac control programs usually took the form of small grants to state health departments and local groups to test screening techniques and to do community education. The USPHS deliberately kept heart disease control programs small in order that they not be perceived as encroaching on the turf of private practitioners.[7]

Public health officials in the pre-Framingham era generally acknowledged that they knew little about the epidemiology of heart disease, knowledge that might ordinarily structure such efforts. The most robust data were from the USPHS-sponsored National Health Survey in 1935–36 in which lay interviewers queried individuals in 700,000 households about the previous year's illness experience. The collected data gave the most accurate picture of cardiovascular disease prevalence and mortality available at that time. But public health officials recognized that the data from this survey, relying on self-reports of illness, were an inadequate foundation for heart disease control. Framingham would later be proposed by the USPHS not only to improve upon these shaky statistics but to test the feasibility of employing more intensive methods of data collection, including physical examinations, to detect heart disease more objectively on a mass scale.[8]

Even though the statistics were shaky, it was obvious to all but a few skeptical voices that CHD incidence was rising. To many lay and medical people, this rise was connected to something in the modern, industrialized world. It was also becoming increasingly evident that CHD was becoming or had become the largest specific cause of adult mortality. But there was little optimism and certainly no concrete knowledge about the prevention of CHD. As late as the mid-1950s, a national commission charged with assessing the state of prevention in chronic disease would devote little space to CHD, noting that the disease "was not preventable at the present time."[9]

On the other hand, in the years prior to 1950 the possibility of preventing CHD was suggested by observations about the geographic variability of CHD, its seemingly rising incidence in the U.S. and Europe, life insurance data pointing to specific associations such as obesity and CHD, and biological evidence that CHD had a particular pathophysiologic basis (atherosclerosis), which suggested it could potentially be prevented and treated. For a few thoughtful observers, such as Ancel Keys, these trends suggested the need for larger-scale epidemiologic studies of CHD. In the 1940s, Keys was a lonely voice arguing that CHD was preventable. Keys collected many epidemiologic observations that associated specific factors in mid-twentieth-century American life with CHD in order to support his application to the USPHS for funds to do a prospective study of "personal characteristics and mode of life" and the development of CHD. Keys sought and received USPHS funding for this study. According to Keys, the USPHS was so impressed with Keys' idea that officials there decided to sponsor a prospective study of their own (Framingham).[10]

Also contributing to the growing interest in conducting epidemiologic studies of CHD were gaps created by the decline in the 1930s and 1940s of an older tradition of clinical speculation about individual predisposition to heart disease.[11] Throughout the previous century, clinicians had offered many sporadic observations about the role of fast-paced modern life, smoking, alcohol, high-fat diet, and heredity in predisposing individuals to angina pectoris, which was typically understood as a chest pain syndrome of uncertain etiology. By 1930, a consensus emerged, especially among the new heart specialists, that angina pectoris and coronary thrombosis were related manifestations of atherosclerotic obstruction of the coronary arteries. As a result, biomedical interest shifted away from individual predisposition to the presumed common anatomic and physiologic disturbances that led to chest pain, thrombosis, and sudden death. Interest in individual predisposition was associated with an older style of general practice, not the new and ascending medical specialties. But many of these ideas persisted in both clinical practice and lay culture and represented the starting point for developing hypotheses about the causes of, and predisposition to, CHD. A more scientifically sound way of investigating these ideas was needed.

In the period before Framingham, many physicians embraced the plausibility of new psychosomatic and constitutional approaches to disease, especially among chronic diseases such as ulcerative colitis, asthma, and hay fever whose pathophysiologic bases were poorly understood and whose clinical course was characterized by unpredictable patterns of exacerbations and remissions. With its new and precise anatomic definition, however, CHD was not a popular target for psychosomatic or constitutional inquiry. Nevertheless, there were a few observers who promoted psychosomatic, holistic, and/or constitutional views of CHD. W. R. Houston, for example, articulated a typical constitution for the individual suffering angina pectoris in the 1920s.[12] As late as 1950, William Stroud could offer a list of constitutional characteristics of the typical patient suffering angina pectoris in his cardiology text.[13]

Against this background, United States Assistant Surgeon General Joseph Mountin proposed in 1947 that the USPHS carry out a large-scale community-based study of CHD. Mountin's proposal initiated the government, academic, and community efforts that resulted in the "Heart Disease Epidemiology Study at Framingham." At its official start in October 1947, Framingham was administered by the Chronic Disease Division of the Bureau of State Services, which mostly channeled federal monies to state and local health departments for community-based chronic disease control programs. Framingham was chosen because of its small size, stable population, proximity to academic resources in Boston, and success as the site for the tuberculosis demonstration project decades earlier.[14]

The initial plan for the study was the result of collaboration between the USPHS, represented by public health officer Gilcin Meadors, the Massachusetts Department of Health, represented by State Health Commissioner Vlado Getting, and Harvard University School of Medicine, represented by David Rutstein, professor of preventive medicine. The initial Framingham proposal called for doing a baseline survey of 5000 or more volunteers who would be reexamined at the end of three to five years with complete exams.[15]

The plan was closer in content to traditional chronic disease control programs than it was to the more ambitious program that would later be devised and implemented. As the Framingham organizers explained to a group of physicians in 1948, the goal of the study was to "determine as early as possible, which persons may develop heart disease, and to bring them under the attention of physicians ... It seems that if we can discover cases early, before actual clinical onset, the patients will have a more useful and productive life and will be able to continue to be supporting citizens in the community, rather than incapacitated, perhaps disabled in some way, and thus a burden upon their families and the communities."[16] As was the case with chronic disease control more generally, Framingham organizers never specified in any detail what medical or other interventions could be offered to cases detected before clinical onset. In some early communications, mention was made of identifying "predisposing factors," but this secondary goal was given less emphasis than devising appropriate techniques for mass screening for heart disease and determining accurate prevalence rates, filling in the gaps left by the earlier USPHS sponsored National Health Survey.[17]

As was also typical of many chronic disease control programs, Framingham was meant to be a laboratory in which better methods of diagnosing early cases of heart disease in a mass setting were developed and tested. Framingham investigators were eager to employ new devices such as the electrokymograph, a device that had been developed by another USPHS cardiac control program, which used both electrical and radiologic information to determine the state of heart function. They hoped these devices would play a diagnostic role for heart disease similar to the role of chest X-rays in tuberculosis control. Framingham planners had no specific plan about how to evaluate these technologies, beyond seeing whether they were feasible to use in a mass setting.[18]

Meadors moved quickly to get the project off the ground. He obtained approval from local hospitals in April 1948, set up an office in July, and began surveying subjects in October. He created many committees, such as those devoted to publicity, industry, business, arrangements, civic organizations, professional matters, and neighborhood organizations. Different types of oversight boards were created, including an advisory committee consisting of prominent Boston cardiologists who were on the executive committee of the American Heart Association. These actions were done to both improve the function of the study as well as to insure community cooperation, and were typical for control programs in the Public Health Service. The first subjects to be surveyed were the community doctors who formed the professional committee, allowing them to feel they were part of the study and preparing them to discuss the program accurately as well as engaging them in recruitment. In the first nine months, hundreds of volunteers were recruited, histories and physicals aimed at diagnosing preexisting heart disease were carried out, and the links with local hospitals, physicians, and community groups were solidified.[19]

Framingham might have remained a study of CHD prevalence and public health techniques for early detection had it not been reorganized and refocused as a consequence of bureaucratic changes within the USPHS. In 1948, Congress established the National Heart Institute (NHI) and included epidemiology within its mission. In July 1949, the founding NHI director, C. J. Van Slyke, looking to fill the empty research portfolio of his newly created institute, took over the Framingham study and engaged statistical experts attached to the new Institute to provide technical support and supervision.[20]

During that summer, Van Slyke, who had developed some interest and experience in epidemiology while working with Surgeon General Thomas Parran in his campaigns against syphilis, consulted with Meadors and suggested an ambitious reformulation of the project, which by then had enrolled some 1000 volunteers. Van Slyke made a number of suggestions that would make Framingham less of a heart control project and more of a descriptive epidemiological study, moving it a step closer to the laboratory and clinical studies that the newly created NHI would soon be funding. Instead of relying on volunteers, Van Slyke urged Meadors to begin again by actively recruiting and selecting a random sample of Framingham adults. Statisticians at NIH recalculated the number of subjects and duration needed to find enough cases of CHD that would allow meaningful comparisons. They suggested that Framingham investigators should recruit some 6000 subjects (after excluding some potential subjects for reasons such as already having coronary heart disease), extend the follow-up period to 20 years, and do complete reexaminations every two years. Under this new plan, only subjects aged 30 or older, as opposed to 20 in the original design, were to be enrolled so that researchers would have a shorter wait for the development of CHD. They also fixed the upper age limit at 60 so that investigators would be able to concentrate on factors that were etiological or predisposing in the not-yet-sick rather than prognostic for those who already had CHD.

Van Slyke also urged that the study collect data on variables that could be easily measured and were similar to information clinicians were used to gathering in typical doctor-patient encounters. Possible causal factors such as diet, occupation, and heredity would be given less emphasis because they were difficult to measure and classify reliably. Van Slyke and Meadors agreed at this time to defer any decision about the difficult job of studying "tension" as a possible causative factor.[21]

In April 1950, Meadors left the study, and a new director, Thomas Dawber, a physician who had previously worked with Van Slyke at the USPHS Marine Hospital in Staten Island, was recruited. By October 1950, Dawber had a large staff in place in Framingham. Dawber understood that Framingham was to be a study of predisposing factors of CHD rather than early detection, testing screening methods, or determining accurate prevalence statistics. He later recalled that Rutstein and the other academics on the advisory board were dissatisfied about the direction the study had originally taken and that local physicians were also skeptical about Meadors because he was not a clinician.[22]

The reorganized, NHI-sponsored Framingham study placed less emphasis on traditional disease control goals. Instead, the new program would try to contribute to an understanding of the fundamental causes of CHD and hypertensive heart disease and to prognostic factors.[23] The study's emphasis had shifted "to the development of the follow up study of normal persons to determine the etiologic and prognostic relationship of various clinical and laboratory procedures to the ultimate development of hypertensive and/or arteriosclerotic heart disease. Prevalence studies, method studies, and the investigation of public health techniques have not been eliminated, but rather will be developed as byproducts of time and funds make such studies possible."[24] In its prospective nature, the redesigned Framingham study had a structure that paralleled a laboratory experiment, even though Framingham involved no intervention.

Prominent Boston cardiologist Paul White was instrumental in encouraging Van Slyke to reconstitute Framingham as a "follow up" study. White was a leading member of the National Heart Advisory Council. He had previously studied in Britain with Sir James McKenzie who had begun a population-based study of heart disease predisposition in his home town of St Andrews, Scotland many years before.[25] In his own lifetime, White had seen coronary thrombosis and angina pectoris go from being rare diagnoses to the most important specific cause of mortality in the western world. It was intuitively obvious to him that some aspect of 20th century life was behind the increased prevalence of the disease.[26]

White had long been a promoter of "follow-up" studies. While a follow-up study is similar to what today we might call a prospective or cohort study, the term had a different connotation in the 1950s and grew out of an older style of elite clinical practice. White's own studies described the long term clinical experience of a group of patients with the same diagnosis or intervention. For example, White and collaborators did a follow up study of the long term prognosis of patients diagnosed with neurocirculatory asthenia (a once commonly diagnosed syndrome characterized by chronic shortness of breath, fatigue, and other symptoms) in which their morbidity and mortality experience was described and compared to those of different reference populations.[27] In this and other follow-up studies, there was typically no predetermined control group. Follow-up studies were initiated by successful clinicians such as White who were in a position to gather information on a large group of patients through time and who also had a particular axe to grind—that close, long term clinical observation, as was only possible by clinicians with large practices, was as useful to the advance of medicine as the laboratory and other experimental studies that by mid-century were becoming essential ingredients of academic success. As applied to Framingham, the term "follow-up study" stressed the importance of clinical experience and observation. White was eager, for example, that Framingham investigate the hunches and observations made by clinicians about CHD, such as its connection to the stresses and strains of fast-paced, modern life.[28]

The changes proposed by Van Slyke, however, were not immediately implemented. What, for example, was going to happen to the many volunteers if the study now called for randomly selected subjects? Dawber felt that the community would react badly if volunteers were asked not to participate and if husbands but not wives were asked to be part of the study.[29] As a result, Framingham investigators continued to study the volunteer group with follow-up visits even though no new volunteers were added to the study after the NHI changes were made. They also decided to sacrifice some scientific generalizability and validity by making the family, not the individual, the unit of randomization.

Framingham investigators also kept and strengthened the community structures and committees that were created when the study was first begun. The study had been sold to the community as having the goals and methods of a cardiac control program, with the implied promise of benefit to individuals and the community. Before the switch to the NHI, this implied promise enabled Framingham investigators to successfully involve the community and recruit volunteers. Framingham investigators now had to explicitly disavow such benefits. "The fact has been stressed that this is a research project," investigators wrote in the early years of the study, "and that when people are examined they have made a contribution to the knowledge of heart disease perhaps which may not benefit them but which it is hoped may benefit some of their grandchildren. Every effort has been made to avoid any appearance of giving service or setting the study up as a service to the community."[30] At the same time, however, investigators continued to capitalize on the community structure and general good feelings that arose from the original emphases. In effect, the community involvement that was part of disease control work was put to different, more purely research-oriented ends. Framingham's later success was thus partly due to the idiosyncrasies of its historical beginnings as a cardiac control program.

Dawber's major concern during the initial reorganization was to keep the two groups most important for the study's success happy—Framingham's private practitioners and the general population. He tried to limit the number and type of diagnostic questions so that subjects would continue to consent to future exams. His model was to make the Framingham exam resemble private practice. Dawber recalled that Framingham subjects were impressed that "it was just like going to a private doctor. You go in there and you are taken care of." This ideal sometimes proved difficult to realize because exams were done by public health service officers who did not have the skills and mind set of the private practitioner and who had to be frequently reminded that Framingham was "not the post office." Dawber kept local practitioners happy by channeling all diagnostic information back to them and by generally treating them with respect. Early on, the Framingham team diagnosed TB in the wife of a prominent practitioner, easing some of the incipient tensions by providing some tangible health benefit, in addition to whatever self-satisfaction comes from contributing to the accretion of knowledge, to a Framingham research subject.[31]

Van Slyke's desire to limit the scope of Framingham's hypotheses to quantifiable, easily measured, clinically apparent factors was also something not immediately acted upon. The Framingham protocol under the NHI, despite Van Slyke's skepticism, retained all kinds of baseline social and psychological data, including variables such as "psychic tone" as well as prior history of what in the 1940s were still thought of as psychosomatic diseases.[32]

In the late 1940s and early 1950s Framingham investigators did not think that they were breaking any new methodological ground with these partially implemented changes. They did not think that Framingham was a novel research study—the first large-scale cohort study of chronic disease. This new identity evolved slowly as a result of the study's reorganization under the newly formed NHI and was perhaps not clearly recognized until the early 1960s. The switch to a follow-up design was not considered methodologically innovative, as the design had been frequently used to better understand prognosis in clinical studies by elite physicians with big practices. While a large government-sponsored follow-up study of individual predisposition to chronic disease was new, the decision to enroll and study a large free-living population was made prior to the idea of a follow-up study. In this sense, Van Slyke and others grafted their new purposes onto a structure that was in place for different reasons.

1951–1970: From near failure to the emergence of risk factors

In 1951, Dawber and colleagues published some results of the initial examinations and the study's rationale for a public health audience.[33] Actual results of the follow-up study would necessarily take a long time to report because even with thousands of subjects there were few new, or "incident," cases of CHD in the first few years that could be used to make inferences about the causes of CHD.

Gradually during the 1950s, Dawber and colleagues simplified the baseline information they collected and abandoned the study of psychological factors, stress, and prior history of psychosomatic dis-eases.[34] Dawber had always been skeptical that "stress" was a useful concept since it was vague and dependent on subjective recollec-tions.[35]

Dawber and his colleagues were similarly skeptical that they could collect reliable data on diet. Diet was therefore largely abandoned de-spite the fact that it was a crucial antecedent to what was to become the most visible tenet of the risk factor mind set—high-fat diet, cho-lesterol, heart disease—and which was center stage in the research of Ancel Keys and others.[36] Thus Framingham investigators in the early 1950s moved away from variables that were subjective and difficult to reliably measure to seemingly more objective quantitative ones.

In the early 1950s, not only did Framingham investigators decide to retain volunteers but they decided in a similar spirit to continue to follow prevalent cases of hypertensive and other forms of heart disease. The Framingham investigators, recognizing that individuals and the community saw the study not merely as a research program but as one that had benefits for its participants, felt that excluding prevalent hypertension cases would be bad public relations. They also recognized that the follow-up data from prevalent cases could be kept separate and be used for making observations about prognosis. This decision led to the inclusion of prevalent cases of hypertension rather than their exclusion from the study—a crucial decision for the nascent risk factor approach. As the study evolved, hypertension was seen less as a defining type of heart pathology than as another antecedent risk.

It was apparent by the early 1950s that the goal of recruiting 6,000 subjects was not feasible. Only 4,494 subjects of the 6,507 invited to participate were recruited despite many efforts (69.1 percent response rate). There was a differential response rate by important variables such as age, sex, and health status. There were also problems of incomplete follow-up among the recruited subjects. Framingham investigators recognized these limitations but understood they were inherent in community studies of heart disease.[37] Dawber had always believed it was a mistake to use an approximately two-thirds sample of the town because many in the remaining third were annoyed that they were not included in the study. He attributed this problem to the lack of understanding of the mind-set of the community by NHI statisticians.[38]

In 1956, nine years after the study was originally conceived, Framingham had attracted little attention within or outside of the medical field. For example, Framingham was mentioned on only a few occasions in the minutes of the National Heart Advisory Council (the chief advisory board for NHI) between 1951 and 1957. Participants in a 1956 national conference on the epidemiology of atherosclerosis and heart disease, sponsored by the NHI and attended by staff in the office of biometry that were working on Framingham, made no mention of Framingham although they periodically emphasized the promise of longitudinally studying apparently healthy populations in time.[39]

In 1956, the NHI decided to review the study. There was a growing apprehension about the project's ultimate success. Nine years after its inception, there were still no publications from the follow-up aspect of the study, the feature that distinguished Framingham from its predecessors. The NHI asked Dr. Thomas Dublin to lead the review. His review was generally positive but noted a few problems. Dublin observed that Framingham investigators had not yet figured out how to study dietary factors. He noted that the staff was very frustrated by the lack of publications and physician ignorance of the study.[40] The staff felt that the fact that "IBM" record keeping was being done in Bethesda was to blame for the dearth of publications. Dublin felt that the problem lay in the lack of an on-site epidemiologist or statistician. He felt the technical advisory board also lacked epidemiological and statistical expertise. He was also concerned about the possible skewed results from the lower-than-expected response rate. He thought that Framingham needed a sociologist or social anthropologist who could help deal with the community-related issues.[41]

Dawber agreed with most of Dublin's findings but resisted the idea of adding a social scientist. Dawber did not have "much confidence that sociologists, social anthropologists, and other similarly labeled persons" would "add anything" to Framingham.[42] He believed that most of the new and important findings in Framingham were not likely to be social or even clinical hypotheses but rather biochemical ones. In addition, Dawber felt that asking subjects about stress or collecting information about their psychological state would seriously damage the study. "If you begin to get too many people in there asking personal questions about their life habits," Dawber recalled about the question of adding social science components to the study, "you are going to kill the whole thing off, so I usually vetoed anything of that kind."[43]

It was not until 1957 that Dawber and colleagues published their first follow-up results, which were the results of the four-year follow-up exam. In general, there were too few outcomes of interest (heart attacks or strokes) to make any strong statements about CHD risk. Nevertheless, analyzing the subset of subjects at highest risk, middle-aged men, Dawber and colleagues found convincing associations among electrocardiograph evidence of left ventricular strain, hypertension, hypercholesterolemia, and weight and later development of what they then called atherosclerotic heart disease.[44]

Dawber was not trained as an epidemiologist, and as Dublin had pointed out, there was no one on site in Framingham who had such expertise. During the time of the study, Dawber and long-time co-investigator William Kannel both pursued graduate work in public health. In the mid-to-late 1950s, there was also little computer support developed for statistical analysis nor were statistical techniques for modeling and understanding multiple influences on outcomes yet developed. The way that the first Framingham results displayed and analyzed multiple interacting factors reflected this state of affairs. In this and other early Framingham reports, investigators usually presented tables of unadjusted incidence data grouped by different variables. Potential interactions were analyzed by stratifying, for example, hypertensives, into separate smoking and nonsmoking groups. Such stratification could allow investigators to determine, for example, whether obesity was directly associated with heart disease or whether its effect was mediated by its impact on other CHD risks, such as high blood pressure.

One specific finding from such stratification in the 1957 report was that the accepted "fact" of obesity as a causal factor in cardiovascular mortality—apparent from life insurance actuarial tables—disappeared when one stratified the population for hypertension. In other words, obesity appeared to exert its effect on cardiovascular mortality by its effect on blood pressure and perhaps other independent risk factors. Only the careful recording of multiple factors antecedent to disease allowed this analysis.[45]

In the late 1950s and early 1960s, Framingham became a much more visible study and interest in preventing CHD grew dramatically. During this period, more follow-up reports from Framingham appeared, but so did others from other places.[46] These reports, along with the growing interest in CHD from external events such as the publicity following President Eisenhower's heart attack in 1956 and the appearance of National Heart Education Council recommendations about screening for heart disease in 1958, led to a greater lay interest in the causes and prevention of the disease.

The earlier frustrations about the limited publications, poor visibility, and statistical naivety of the Framingham study were quickly overcome. A bibliography from the National Heart Institute of original publications based on Framingham data lists 1 publication in 1957, 1 in 1958, 4 in 1959, 1 in 1960, 5 in 1961, 14 in 1962, 7 in 1963, 4 in 1964, 7 in 1965, 9 in 1966, 13 in 1967, 6 in 1968, 10 in 1969, and 10 in 1970. In the 1970s, there were on average 19 publications each year; in the 1980s, 25 publications per year. In 1990 alone, there were 50 original publications by Framingham researchers.[47]

By the early 1960s, the findings of Framingham investigators reached a wide general and medical audience. The early results were influential in the construction of a canon of prospectively determined risks for later development of CHD: hypertension, elevated serum cholesterol, EKG findings of left ventricular hypertrophy, male sex, family history of premature CHD, and smoking. These results appeared in popular magazines, public health journals, general medicine journals, insurance trade journals, geriatrics journals, nutrition journals, cardiology journals, other subspecialty journals, government publications, proceedings of scientific meetings, and medical throwaways. Framingham investigators actively worked to reach a wide audience with their results. According to Kannel, "we would publish almost anywhere." Unlike mainstream epidemiologists who "got the most gratification out of a good model," Framingham investigators were trained as clinicians and had a message — "what kills these people" — that they wanted to deliver to clinicians and public health officials.[48]

The term "risk factor" first appeared in a Framingham publication in 1961.[49] The expression quickly took off. By 1965, the term was used in most heart disease epidemiology publications and in most lay magazine and newspaper coverage of research into heart disease epidemiology. The term was used without definition or special emphasis, suggesting that there was little consciousness that the term was new or suggested any new conception of the disease.

Framingham both influenced and exemplified the emerging risk factor approach as it contributed to redefining the identity and scope of public health. In 1964, Dawber argued that data from studies such as Framingham formed the basis for a new preventive medicine to be distinguished from both traditional public health and clinical practice. "Preventive medicine," he proclaimed, "is largely the prevention of disease or disability through individual effort, both by the physician and patient."[50] The implication of Dawber's distinction was both bureaucratic and ideological. Unlike public health activities that were either independent of (e.g., improved sanitation) or seemingly in competition with (e.g., free tuberculosis clinics) traditional fee-for-service private medical practice, the new preventive medicine was to take place in the offices of physicians in private medical practice.[51]

Ultimately, the results of Framingham and other studies were packaged as a series of discrete risk factors that clinicians could easily uncover by taking a medical history, conducting a physical examination, and ordering some laboratory tests. Moreover, some risk factors could be treated by medicines prescribed by doctors or modified by behavioral changes suggested by them. Framingham, starting out as a public health initiative in an era in which private practitioners were distrustful of public health efforts, had co-opted this opposition by producing knowledge in a way that respected the needs of, and was useful to, physicians in private practice. Throughout the study, for example, no therapeutics were ever given to the subject, and information on individual subjects was always directed to the patient's private practitioner. Framingham thus contributed to a new risk-factor-based preventive medicine in which traditional public health ends (primary prevention of disease) were to be achieved by physicians in private practice.

The scientific basis for this new preventive medicine was Framingham-like risk factors that were studied and expressed using new multivariate statistics. Multivariate statistical techniques were gradually assimilated into the Framingham study beginning in the late 1950s. According to Kannel, many of these techniques saw their first biomedical use in the Framingham study.[52] Some Framingham research publications represented advances in statistical technique as evidenced by their publication in statistical journals.[53] Framingham investigators had joined forces with NIH-based biometricians to deploy newly devised multiple logistic regression techniques to model multiple influences on cardiac outcomes simultaneously and to build models by which their relative and absolute effect on CHD could be quantified. The end results were complicated risk factor equations, in which an individual's risk of CHD could be quantitatively expressed.

These multivariate statistical techniques were not employed without reservations. Dawber was very suspicious of them, arguing both that they were an attempt to get something (inferences) from nothing (inadequate sample size) by using complicated mathematical techniques.[54] Furthermore, the type of stratification used by Dawber in presentations to actuaries and clinicians in the late 1950s and early 1960s made more intuitive sense than multivariate statistics and did not require the audience for Framingham to have a sophisticated statistical background. The new multivariate models were often as opaque and unintelligible as their conclusions were precise and mathematical.

The multivariate model allowed multiple, in theory unlimited, influences to be tested against and along with one another. This contributed to the widespread use of the term "multifactorial" to describe the etiology of CHD and other diseases—and to skepticism.[55] As mentioned earlier, the often open-ended (i.e., not hypothesis-driven) search for the multifactorial etiology of CHD in the 1950s aroused the skepticism of the external reviewers of the project. The use of a variety of changing dependent and independent variables led to suspicions that the study was not "scientific," because investigators might tinker with the data to see what associations worked and then afterwards declare them to be motivating hypotheses. This open-endedness of both causal factors and outcomes would later become a hallmark of modern risk factor epidemiology, and made that much more doable, if no less scientifically suspect, by the use of computerized analysis.

Kannel and Castelli would later recall that "anything that you could measure that became associated with a higher rate of heart attack or stroke later in life became known as a risk factor."[56] The new statistical techniques and computers made finding and studying these associations much easier. Thus risk factors increasingly took on an empirical and ad hoc identity that invited skepticism about particular claims, the meaning of quantitative risk equations, and clinical models built on such equations (e.g., the risk disk, a bedside tool for computing a patient's chances of experiencing a cardiac event from Framingham-like risk factors).[57] Given the ability to model almost any feature of an individual alongside other risk factors, it is not surprising that some observers have studied ear lobe patterns and palm creases as possible risk factors for CHD. which seem more like fortune teller signs than fundamental causes of the disease.[58]

The precise and quantitative relationships among the multiple risk factors sometimes gave the appearance that a true predictive science of predisposition to disease had emerged. Framingham investigators generally checked these deterministic ambitions. One problem in imputing causality from association was that risk factors were presumed to lead to coronary atherosclerosis, yet there was no good way to measure atherosclerosis directly in an epidemiological study. The endpoints that they used—coronary death, heart attack, and angina pectoris—were only indirectly related to coronary atherosclerosis. Pathological processes besides atherosclerosis, such as platelet stickiness, contributed to coronary thrombosis. Because these other processes had been both poorly understood and identified, there had to be certain indeterminacy in risk factor associations. Angina pectoris, which had essentially become by 1950 a chest pain syndrome in someone with suspected or proven coronary pathology, had not typically been understood as a direct consequence of any single, specific pathology because individuals varied in their pain thresholds, experience of pain, and in their health-reporting and health-seeking behavior. This issue has repeatedly appeared in discussions about why women have been more frequently diagnosed with angina pectoris than men. Finally, observers have acknowledged that there might well be a degree of irresolvable uncertainty in precisely understanding who develops clinically-evident CHD because of the multitude of idiosyncratic influences operating at the level of the individual, no matter how detailed our knowledge of pathophysiology becomes.[59]

The seemingly precise and quantitative logistic regression formulas that resulted from the new techniques had a verisimilitude to causal explanations, i.e., for a given individual, cardiac risk was a precise function of blood pressure times a constant, plus the number of affected relatives under 60 times a constant, plus the number of pack-years of cigarette smoking times a constant, etc. In a similar way, the statistical concept of independence was frequently equated with the notion of fundamental cause.

But the equation of statistical independence and fundamental cause and the resulting implication that the identification of independent influences would allow targeted scientific interventions was and remains problematic. A risk factor that makes some independent contribution to CHD may not be the most important point of clinical or public health intervention. For example, while Framingham investigators were able to discern that obesity was not an independent risk factor for CHD, while hypertension was, it may very well be that interventions aimed at reducing weight might be preferable to solely identifying individuals with hypertension and lowering their blood pressure with medications. Obesity may be more easily recognized and monitored, more closely tied to other health problems, and more easily in-

fluenced by changing social norms and advertising than an independent factor such as hypertension.

Framingham investigators felt that the study not only contributed
to a new preventive medicine, but gave more scientific power to epidemiology. In 1963, Dawber, Kannel, and Lyell argued that epidemiology was not only the study of how disease is distributed, but also an
"approach to the unraveling of secrets pertaining to the development
of disease through the identification of factors which are directly or
indirectly associated with the disease."[60] Framingham's success meant
that epidemiological methods were more than a source of hunches for,
stepsister to, or hypothesis generator for laboratory investigation.[61]

Yet another way Framingham contributed to, and exemplified, the
risk factor approach is its influence on the rhetoric of risk and disease, especially with regards to the meaning of terms such as "normal" and concepts such as the threshold risk for disease. The finding
of a continuous level of risk for serum cholesterol, even at low serum
levels, suggested that the notion of "normal" needed some modification. As Dawber and Kannel put it, "It is important to recognize that
in the United States population, there is no level of serum cholesterol
which can be called 'normal' in the sense that such a level implies absence of risk of CHD. There is no level at which the risk takes a sudden
rise."[62] The meaning of "abnormal" shifted from a dangerous level of
smoking, serum cholesterol, and hypertension to something relative
and unfixed. Thresholds have generally provided a comforting conception of risk for individuals, clinicians, and epidemiologists by lib-
erating judgments about risk and normality from the complexities
of an unbounded relativism. However, such thresholds were rarely
found in Framingham or other studies of CHD risk. Instead, public
policy makers would have to construct them based on economic, feasibility, and political concerns, and since they were so constructed,
they have always been suspect and subject to controversy.

Another problem arising from the meaning of epidemiological
associations has sometimes been framed as the epidemiological or
policy makers' paradox.[63] On the one hand, individuals at highest risk
for CHD were those who had extreme values of many risk factors. On
the other hand, the great majority of individuals with CHD had only
modest elevations of a few or single risk factors — or no risk factors. As

a consequence of this "paradox," the clinical and public health strategy that leads to identifying and treating those individuals at highest risk may only have a small impact on the population's health.

Despite the success of the Framingham study, the NIH moved in the late 1960s to close down the project. Kannel believed that laboratory investigators at the NIH, such as prominent kidney researcher Robert Berliner, who had long resented the intramural commitment of funds as well as the publicity accorded to Framingham, were able to take advantage of the Nixon budget cuts in federal research spending to propose cutting the program. Framingham had been anomalous in its length and its geographical organization—a supposed intramural program (one directly contracted and administered by NIH staff) whose biometric analysis was carried out in Bethesda while the study was in Framingham. The decision to cut Framingham was itself unusual as it was not an institute-level determination (i.e., NHI) but a central NIH one.[64]

The explicit reasons given for the decision to terminate included that the original twenty-year follow-up plan was nearing completion, the study had done its job, and budget cutting was the order of the day. Framingham investigators, however, did not accept the decision quietly. William Kannel was eventually censured by NIH director James Watt for lobbying for its continuation.[65] Paul White tried to influence the decision by appealing to Nixon.[66] Framingham and Boston newspapers and community activists started a public relations campaign to influence Washington. As Kannel recalled, this publicity probably caused the NIH administration to dig in its heels.[67] Giving in to public pressure was understood as putting politics into what should be a scientific decision.

The public relations campaign, along with other efforts and pressures, generated enough interest to allow Framingham to continue under other auspices. Community and corporate donations were solicited, and Boston University took over the management of the study. One ironic consequence of the NIH decision to close Framingham was the increased cost of the study for the NIH in extramural support and in meeting its commitment to provide statistical support.[68] As an extramural program, receiving funding by NIH and other sources, the study has continued through the present.

Conclusion

Framingham began as a cardiac control program similar to many older TB public health campaigns and slowly evolved into what came to be seen as the first large-scale cohort study of chronic disease. There was never a single moment in which the novel methodological aspects were invented or recognized. Framingham investigators tacked this way and that in response to the influence of its changing institutional base, the needs of its various supporters and audiences, and new conceptual and practical tools.

Framingham both helped shape and embodied a new approach to individual predisposition to disease that was individualistic, precise, quantitative, and as a result generally viewed as more scientific than earlier approaches. By choosing to study individual parameters rather than group ones, Framingham investigators contributed to a risk factor approach that was more *individualistic* than social, environmental, or holistic. An estimate of the number of cigarettes smoked by Framingham subjects could easily be entered into risk factor equations, but the influence of tobacco advertising or price subsidies could not. Although Framingham rhetoric stressed that it was a community study, in one sense the 5,000 subjects were studied as a collection of individuals rather than as part of a social framework. The study population was not compared to other communities or even characterized in social terms beyond income and education. As mentioned earlier, what was initially attractive about Framingham as a community was its homogeneity.

Framingham's near-exclusive focus on individuals was not premeditated or driven by ideology. It resulted from a number of factors, especially investigator desire that the study look as much like a clinical experiment as possible. Framingham investigators hoped to earn the study a legitimate place in the NHI, where their laboratory investigator peers were poised to criticize Framingham from its earliest beginnings as data dredging, overly ambitious, and interminable—and who dropped the program in the late 1960s. The individualist focus of Framingham also resulted from investigator desire to use data and variables that could be easily understood and used by the clinician in a busy fee-for-service practice.

Critics of the risk factor approach have pointed out that risk factors are not randomly distributed in the population. Rather, they are determined by social and political factors that are the root causes of bad health more generally. According to these critics, the focus on finding those individuals with high blood pressure, high cholesterol, and glucose intolerance and giving them medicines means that we are not addressing the social and political status quo, which encourages tobacco production and distribution and social conditions, including poor education and housing, drug use, and breakdown of the family, that have led to unhealthy behaviors such as high-fat diet and lack of physical exercise.[69]

Framingham investigators recognized the limitations of focusing their study on factors that operate at the level of the individual. According to Kannel, the social and economic factors that might explain or support changes in an individual's diet, sedentariness, and smoking habits were very important, but not the focus of Framingham. They were someone else's problem.[70]

Framingham investigators contributed to a new quantitative, individualistic, and seemingly more scientific approach to individual predisposition to disease. This new approach allowed both lay and medical people to reconsider and reformulate ideas about CHD that had been widely discussed before the ascendancy of modern cardiology and its focus on anatomic and physiologic disorders. For example, the notion that "type A personality" was a CHD risk factor in effect reformulated much older ideas about stress and CHD.[71] The results of studies such as Framingham gave new life and scientific respectability to much older ideas and interests, especially the idea that individuals were responsible for their diseases.

The risk factor approach has been appealing for a number of reasons. It potentially gives individuals a road map with which to negotiate among different behavioral and lifestyle choices on the way to achieving health. It also provides a consoling framework with which to minimize the frightening randomness of disease. Finally, it provides a sanctioned vehicle, in a secular era, with which to say certain individuals and groups are doing the right thing and others the wrong thing (e.g., overeating, smoking, not taking medicines, never exercising).[72]

While many of these appealing features of the risk factor approach seem timeless and universal, the approach is at the same time a product of specific developments and characteristics of late twentieth-century American medicine and culture more generally: the rise of government-sponsored, centralized "big ticket research" and medical specialization; the high prestige of laboratory science and laboratory scientists; the growing awareness of the limitations of reductionist models of disease; the uncertain health benefits attributable to specific medical interventions; the development and diffusion of computer-assisted multivariate statistical techniques; and the perceived need to make public health research relevant and useful for clinicians in fee-for-service practice. It is a style of conceptualizing, talking about, and intervening in what individuals bring to disease that evolved incrementally and without much medical or lay awareness of its novelty or historical importance.

The Framingham study evolved incrementally in response to a number of micro- and macrodevelopments, similar if not identical to many of those that determined the emergence of the risk factor approach. Contemporary medical and lay ambivalence about these new approaches and methods, reflected daily in so many ways—from mass media coverage of scientific studies "proving" that yesterday's healthy behaviors have become today's risks to policy conflicts over how and whether to screen for this or that disease—directly follows from the often contradictory and competing influences that have shaped the history of late twentieth-century epidemiologic science and our styles of explaining health and disease.

5

Gardasil: A vaccine against cancer and a drug to reduce risk

Merck began its "One Less" advertising campaign for Gardasil, its vaccine against human papillomavirus (HPV), in 2006, not long after Gardasil received U.S. Food and Drug Administration approval.[1] In a widely broadcast television advertisement, girls and young women of different ethnicities and apparently different socioeconomic backgrounds chant "I want to be one less ... one less statistic." One woman says, "Gardasil is the only vaccine that may help protect you against the four types of HPV that may cause 70 percent of cervical cancer," and another (older) woman warns of side effects.[2] Viewers of these advertisements might have wondered why, if Gardasil was "the only cervical cancer vaccine," its name had to be endlessly repeated. Some might also have pondered the uncertain efficacy introduced by the repeated use of "may" and just how likely they were to be one of the "thousands of women" who develop cervical cancer each year.

People looking at a print advertisement for Gardasil that appeared around the same time were offered a different rationale than becoming one less cancer statistic. This advertisement suggested that Gardasil allowed the consumer to evade the *risk* of contracting HPV. "She won't have to tell him she had HPV ... because she doesn't."[3]

This chapter explores the details and implications of Gardasil's co-construction as a vaccine against cancer and as a proprietary drug that promises reduction and control of individual risk. One might immediately question whether Gardasil is any different from some vaccines introduced in the past, which had elements of public goods as well as of commodities and which aimed to benefit populations as well as individual vaccine consumers. While these continuities exist, Gardasil has entered American medicine and society at a time when intervening in individual risk has become central to the health care economy, medical and lay understandings of efficacy, and the experience of health and disease. These changed features, as they relate to Gardasil and generally to health risk interventions, are sometimes difficult to appreciate because researchers, public health officials, drug manufacturers, and clinicians have blurred the border between risk and disease and have appropriated older rationales and the language of traditional clinical interventions and public health. They have often done so intentionally and for narrow, self-interested purposes.

So although Gardasil is not a completely novel vaccine and the controversies it has sparked are not unprecedented, it has appeared under new circumstances in American medicine and society that have shaped every aspect of its development, architecture, marketing, and reception. These circumstances, described below from the medical literature, media accounts, advertisements, and policy deliberations available to the public, can help explain some of the widespread ambivalence Gardasil has evoked, especially the gap between the promise of effectively preventing cancer and many Americans' weariness with the introduction of yet another risk-reducing commodity.[4]

Gardasil's meaning has also been influenced by an epidemiological reality far different from the one in which many of the most effective vaccines against epidemic and endemic childhood diseases (e.g., polio and measles) were introduced. Because of the success of earlier vaccine programs and other developments, the potential targets for new vaccines are generally less prevalent conditions. Many new potential target diseases have other means of prevention and are treatable if contracted. This diminishing potential population benefit constitutes a void that can be filled by a greater focus on individual risk.

My argument is not that Gardasil is more a drug against risk than a vaccine. It is both of these things, Janus faced, with one identity featured more prominently than the other depending on the context of use. The class of immunological interventions we call vaccines is a very heterogeneous category, whose prototype and namesake, the smallpox vaccine, is no longer in active service. The prototypical vaccine is directed against a specific, prevalent, serious, and communicable infectious disease. It reproduces the lifelong immunity given by natural infection. Because of its high efficacy in individuals, the prototypical vaccine contributes to herd immunity: it interrupts the spread of disease by reducing the number of susceptible individuals.[5] The prototypical vaccine thus serves population goals, not just individual ones, and thereby provides a major rationale for public funding, coercive rules such as those requiring vaccination for entry into school, and calls for universal administration.

In practice, many vaccines now and in the past have strayed from this idealized notion of a vaccine. Typhoid vaccine's immunity is so short-lived that it is mostly used to protect tourists. Pneumococcal vaccine targets many but not all of the infection-causing bacterial subtypes. Tetanus vaccine is aimed at a noncommunicable disease. Influenza vaccine is designed anew each year to respond to antigenic drift and the perceived danger of different influenza strains. Bacillus Calmette-Guérin (BCG) vaccine offers only partial immunity for a disease that does not normally induce immunity. To say that Gardasil is not a prototypical vaccine makes it like many other vaccines.

Risk, causality, HPV, and cervical cancer

Risk is central to the definition and diagnosis of HPV infection and cervical cancer and the causal links between them. HPV types are defined quantitatively and probabilistically as having a less than 10 percent difference in nucleate assays. They have been named (in this case, numbered) by their order of discovery. As a result, the ontology of any particular HPV type is necessarily problematic, as are causal claims based upon them, for example, the claim that HPV types 16 and 18 are *the cause* of 70 percent of cervical cancer.

Infection by one of these HPV types, however necessary a condition in the causal chain, does not by itself lead to cancer. HPV infection is common; cervical cancer is rare. Other risk factors that have emerged from epidemiological studies include smoking, having multiple HPV-type infections, being older, and being coinfected with other sexually transmitted diseases such as chlamydia and genital herpes. These risk factors explain little of the population variance but serve as a reminder that we do not understand precisely the etiology of cervical cancer at either the individual or the population level.[6]

Although the mechanisms by which HPV infection leads to cancer have been more directly observed than almost any other carcinogen-cancer relationship, the carcinogenic role of particular HPV types is nevertheless dependent on the probabilities that specific regions of HPV DNA will survive host immune reaction, integrate with cervical epithelial DNA, survive DNA repair, and lead to clonal autonomy and immortality. Chance and poorly understood ecological factors (immune or otherwise) not only influence these processes but also may or may not keep at bay a particular cancer clone fully capable of growth and metastasis, which is yet another reason that prediction of the clinical course of patients from their cervical biopsies has long been difficult.[7]

During a regulatory hearing for Gardasil, a Merck representative conceded that our knowledge about the causal connection between high-risk HPV types and cervical cancer was necessarily indirect and open to revision. "There was—there isn't any marker that says, you know, okay, here's an HPV 16. It is glomming right onto the cell and causing it to be malignant, if you know what I mean. Just the strong associations between these things and the fact that persistent HPV 16 infection is highly likely to cause disease and the association with 16 is particularly relevant for cervical cancer, 18 for adenocarcinoma and so on."[8]

Despite these uncertainties, the evidence for the causal link between HPV and cervical cancer is tighter than for almost any other causal association in cancer.[9] HPV infection has been directly observed and visualized within various precursor lesions and pathological specimens of full-blown invasive cervical cancer. There is also very precise knowledge of which HPV DNA regions seem to be most transformative and get incorporated in clones destined to become cancerous. Additionally, the role HPV is understood to play in cancer transformation makes adaptive sense when looked at from the perspective of the virus (viruses that are successful at integrating into the cervical cell genome and at inducing immortality will produce more progeny).[10]

"Scientific" efficacy of cervical cancer vaccines is uncertain

Despite the highly plausible observations linking HPV to cervical cancer, not only does causality remain contested but the strength of the causal association does not necessarily predict what will happen when a causal factor is removed. On ethical and statistical grounds (i.e., the numbers of subjects and the time needed to measure a significant change in cancer mortality), there will never be a randomized placebo-controlled trial of HPV immunization with cervical cancer mortality as an endpoint. This is an old problem. For similar reasons, there has never been a randomized controlled trial of Pap smears with this endpoint.[11] Our belief that the widespread use of the Pap smear has led to the decline in cervical cancer mortality rests on a set of assumptions about the natural history of precancerous cervical abnormalities and the effectiveness of their "early" removal.[12] Using the declining cervical cancer mortality to support the efficacy of Pap smears is problematic, if for no other reason than that this decline preceded the introduction of widespread Pap screening.[13]

So instead of cervical cancer incidence and mortality, clinical trials of HPV vaccine efficacy have had to make do with using HPV-type-specific cytological abnormalities as endpoints. The principal evidence establishing Gardasil's efficacy has been the reduction of different cervical abnormalities and putative cancer "precursors" that contain HPV 16 and 18 infections within them. Using this measure, Gardasil is nearly 100 percent effective.

It remains unclear, however, whether reducing these types of abnormalities will translate into reduced cervical cancer incidence and mortality. To understand why extrapolating from such limited endpoints may ultimately be misleading, consider one scenario. Reduction in the incidence of high-risk HPV types 16 and 18 through vaccination may result in a higher incidence of other HPV types. We do not know whether types 16 and 18 are intrinsically more virulent than other types or are only more successful at infecting individuals relative to other types. This is a nontrivial issue. To the degree that type-specific associations with cancer are due to their greater success at infection in competition with other types rather than an inherent capacity for harm, the theoretical concern about the dangers of type replacement mentioned during regulation hearings and elsewhere is real. Will vaccines in effect select for different dominant HPV types, which may turn out to have a much higher pathogenicity than previously appreciated? Such a subtype replacement phenomenon may be occurring with currently used multivalent pneumococcal vaccines, which like HPV vaccines contain some but not all disease-causing subtypes.[14]

Complicating any determination of the possible impact of Gardasil on cervical cancer are the possible effects of Gardasil on the detection and meaning of cervical cancer and even on sexual behavior. Will the vaccine lead to more or less cervical cancer screening and be efficacious by this indirect route? Will there be a shift in cases from squamous cell carcinoma to adenocarcinoma of the cervix? Will coincident HPV infection or genomic integration become part of the case definition of cervical cancer, leading to new types of cases that are necessarily influenced by HPV screening and Gardasil administration?

But my aim is not to simply fan the skeptical fire. In the case of Gardasil, there are many reasons to hope that there will be significant positive population benefits. Yet our current ignorance and the general unpredictable nature of ecological and evolutionary developments are real. The effects of massive immunization campaigns on populations are complex and difficult to predict. Net long-term (as in decades or generations) effects are even more unclear and have provided fodder for vaccine skeptics. These uncertainties underscore what is apparent from the history of other vaccination programs (see note 4). They are massive population experiments and should be treated as such. This uncertain population impact is one of the main reasons that promoters of Gardasil have appealed to additional types of efficacy besides received notions of objective and material improvement in the morbidity and mortality of individuals and populations.

Efficacy as risk reduction and control

Gardasil has been constructed and marketed to have an impact on an individual's experience of risk. The vaccine promises to control fears and bring some relief from feelings of randomness, shame, and stigma. This rationale is not trumpeted. Highlighting too boldly individual risk control can potentially undermine the more scientific and idealized views of efficacy through which Gardasil and many other products are rationalized and by which they are legitimated and approved within the scientific and regulatory worlds.

Let's begin with a fantasy of Gardasil's initial development and marketing. This fantasy cannot easily be checked against reality because the negotiations behind the launching of new drugs are shrouded in privacy. Someone at Merck, GlaxoSmithKline, or elsewhere perhaps woke up one morning and realized that the firm's prestigious, effective, morally upright but only marginally profitable vaccine business was looking strangely like their drugs-for-individualized-risk division, the company's most profitable.

Jeremy Greene has described the pharmaceutical industry's skillful use of clinical trials to simultaneously establish efficacy and promote new types of risky targets for drugs. Greene begins his narrative at a 1957 meeting of the American Drug Manufacturer's Association in which an industry representative reflected on the paradoxical market impact of the industry's most obvious success—the production and marketing of antibiotics. Antibiotics' success at curing infectious disease had the effect of limiting the industry's market. No profitable industry's business model would want to create products that completely consumed demand for them. The representative called for a new paradigm for drug development and marketing. In 1957 this representative could only imagine the outlines of another paradigm in which drugs would grow rather than shrink their market. In following years, the pharmaceutical industry developed and marketed risk-reducing drugs and a new probabilistic concept of efficacy as risk reduction.[15]

Unlike the antibiotics market, the market for risk-reducing drugs is potentially the whole population, and the duration of use could span a consumer's entire life. The evidence for this new "at-risk" monetary and moral economy is all around us yet is often framed in ways that obscure what is happening. While policy debates raged around Medicare financing of prescription drugs at the end of the twentieth century, few analysts were discussing the fact that the elderly, like everyone else, were largely taking "risk-reducing" drugs (see chapter 9). Observers of Merck's Vioxx debacle, retold as a morality and liability story in various courtroom, media, and policy forums, usually pay only passing attention to the fact that Merck definitively proved or stumbled onto the up-to-then debated cardiovascular risk in the midst of a clinical trial to see if Vioxx might reduce colon cancer risk, the ultimate rationale for a mass-marketed risk-reducing pharmaceutical. It is intrinsic, not accidental, that the attempt to find a mass risk-reducing identity for drugs can backfire. The Vioxx debacle illustrates the characteristic "easy come, easy go" problem when efficacy is constructed as individualized risk reduction. Risk-reducing drugs are especially vulnerable to data suggesting that they carry their own risks. How can one aggressively sell peace of mind, insurance, and freedom from fear when the very same product shows evidence of producing further risks? Others have pointed out the American cultural aversion to imposed risk.[16]

Risk-reducing pharmaceuticals promise to eliminate or control the fears, discomfort, and hassles associated with risk. It is the *experience* of risk, not only the objective, specific danger, that is the object of elimination, control, and reduced hassle (see chapter 3).

All of these general features of our new "risk reduction as efficacy" paradigm are operative in contemporary attempts to control and contain cervical cancer risk. A large fraction of the adult female population gets annual Pap screening.[17] Close to three million of these women annually will be told they have an abnormality. Some will only have repeat studies, but others will undergo procedures such as colposcopy and biopsy and perhaps live for a time with the suspicion or frank diagnosis of cervical cancer or one of the many associated precancerous diagnoses. If tested and found positive for HPV (as part of the Pap test, following a Pap abnormality, or because of a wart), they will be told—depending on whether typical testing was done and what the results were—that they are capable of transmitting this cancer- and/or wart-causing virus to their sexual partners and that even condoms might not be fully protective.

It is against this intervened-in and experienced risk state that Gardasil's efficacy for individuals must be understood. The vaccine may result in one less cervical cancer victim, but it promises every consumer the chance to evade or reduce the risk of infection with cancer- or wart-causing HPV strains. This risk state is made more palpable by being communicable and embodied. In this latter quality it is like so many other noninfectious but worrisome precancerous entities.[18]

I referred earlier to the message that appeared in a print advertisements, "She won't have to tell him she had HPV . . . because she
doesn't." This message more overtly sells Gardasil's efficacy at evading or controlling the risk experience, which in the case of HPV is the
stigma and worry attached to harboring a sexually transmissible disease that can lead to warts and cancer. I have had numerous patients
and students over the years express their worry, shame, and confusion
about what to do after being told that they had an HPV infection. They
were understandably worried about infecting others with a cancer-
causing virus and feared uncomfortable discussions and negotiations
at extremely awkward moments.[19]

I know parents who have urged their daughters to get the HPV vaccine less out of fear that they would develop cervical cancer than to
prevent or minimize the anxiety, shame, and guilt associated with
HPV risk and to avoid the tests and interventions that follow an abnormal Pap smear.[20] In sum, the desire to avoid the experience of embodied risk may be a significant driver of the initial Gardasil demand,
especially among the more affluent. It also helps explain why and how
the vaccine/drug was marketed to middle-class women, priced high,
and sold as a consumer choice, by advertisements similar in tone and
content to the ones for many risk-reducing drugs such as statins. Although at low risk of cervical cancer, more affluent individuals generally have a great deal of knowledge and experience with abnormal
screening tests and their psychological and other consequences.

Merck has not pushed this "risk/fear control" rationale very explicitly in print and television commercials. Fear and avoidance of shame
work better as subliminal messages. The appeal of control needs little
emphasis once fear and other negative consequences of a risk state
have been effectively communicated. Made too explicit, such messages are easily exposed and ridiculed as fear mongering.[21] However,
evading the sexual aspects of HPV transmission and the resulting
stigma can itself be open to criticism and invite parody.

Cancer risk reduction is perhaps too serious a target for parody. But
another direct-to-consumer-marketed product, Valtrex—an antiviral
medicine used to treat herpes infections, which similarly promises to
protect people from sexual transmission of a disease in a highly probabilistic fashion—has invited many parodies. In one Valtrex advertisement, seen frequently in our home, different (presumably sexual)
partners of various ages and ethnicity (but not same-sex partners)

face the screen. One says "I have herpes." The other says, "And I don't." Voice-overs and different actors then give a litany of side effects and warnings of limited efficacy.[22] This advertisement has spawned parodies that make fun of the sanitary and inexplicit way the stigma and fear of sexual transmission and impurity are presented as well as the many hedges about the vaccine's safety and efficacy.[23] In a typical parody, the affected partner straightforwardly announces that she or he has herpes, just as in the real advertisement. But there is no smiling and understanding unaffected partner. Upon hearing that his or her partner has herpes, the unaffected partner hurls curses ("you whore"), and violence sometimes ensues. Behind the black humor is a warning to Merck and other drug manufacturers to keep the control of sexually transmitted disease at a distance from products that can be sold in a more highbrow way.[24]

Vaccine composition, architecture, and cost: Strategies for maximizing risk and benefit

HPV vaccines are composed of ingenious virus-like particles (VLPs). Type-specific viral proteins of the L1 class produced by recombinant genetic technology organize themselves into VLPs that strongly resemble the wild-type HPV virus but contain no DNA. Gardasil consists of four of these VLPs, each derived from different HPV serotypes. Two of the types (16 and 18) are associated with the development of cervical cancer, the other two with warts.[25] In what sense is this combination VLP vaccine a drug against individual risk?

The rationale and function of this particular mix of VLPs is similar to the way a stock portfolio or mutual fund works to manage risk and benefit. This combination product has been designed to reach a reasonable trade-off between the probable benefits of immunity to multiple HPV types and the risk that including noncarcinogenic targets might dilute the immunity to the cancer-causing ones as well as adding costs and side effects. Like a stock portfolio or a bundled set of risky investments, Gardasil diversifies and reduces risk and appeals to multiple market segments (people who want cancer protection and people who don't want warts), making the drug more palatable and giving it a large market. In particular, the addition of the wart-causing capsids expands the drug's target market to boys and men, building on the less compelling (in terms of numbers impacted and what can marketed without controversy) rationales for the male market such as preventing HPV-associated cancers in men such as anal carcinoma. Overall, this composite identity increased the benefit side of the risk-benefit equation for individuals taking the vaccine and thereby helped to ease the drug's passage through regulatory bottlenecks in which cost-effectiveness considerations from the individual consumer's perspective were paramount.

At about $300 for the three immunizations, Gardasil is currently priced out of the ballpark of cost-effectiveness associated with mandated, universally recommended, and often subsidized vaccines. It is similarly too expensive for mass use in the developing world, leading to controversial subsidized programs discussed in chapter 8. Merck is presumably trying to recover its development costs and make a profit by selling the vaccine at a high price to a limited segment of affluent and well-insured, worried Americans, especially while it remained the sole HPV vaccine. Later, when pressures from competitors and price reductions are sought by government mass purchase, it might be a better strategy to lower the price and widen the market, as has been done with other vaccines.

Priced in this way, however, Merck's initial marketing gives preference to Gardasil's impact on individuals rather than the population. A similar logic lies behind the decision to initially seek approval to give the vaccine only to girls. Cost-effectiveness analysis has shown a much lower marginal cost-effectiveness when boys are added to the population mix. This conclusion is more easily reached when the cost of the vaccine is high and by the use of assumptions and econometric techniques that do not measure herd immunity.

Manufactured as a risk-reducing pill

As a recombinant DNA product, Gardasil's material reality and its production more closely resemble pharmaceuticals such as Humulin and many new cancer and immunological therapies such Herceptin, Interferon, and Remicaid than traditional vaccines. Vaccines as technologies and products have historically emerged from the companies or divisions of pharmaceutical companies that make biologicals. In the early twentieth century, these firms often made serums and antitoxins using live animals. The production of many of the vaccines that replaced serums and toxins similarly involved live whole organisms, eggs, tissue cultures, and so forth. Innovation and production involved a great deal of knowledge about managing and manipulating living organisms, often on a mass scale—hundreds of thousands of eggs, chickens, and other living organisms. The emergence of recombinant DNA technology may mean that this era of biologicals is coming to an end.[26]

One consequence of this new recombinant DNA production is that Gardasil and other similarly produced vaccines may find it much easier to ensure patent protection—and thus higher profits for patent holders—than the older biologicals. In the era of biologicals, there were often many different and difficult-to-specify ways to isolate immunogenic material from infectious organisms and to attenuate them while preserving immunogenicity. Once the possibility of developing a vaccine had been demonstrated, different biological techniques could be used to develop similarly effective products. These differences in production made patent protection for vaccines-as-biologicals more difficult than for the vaccines currently produced by recombinant DNA technology.

Furthermore, the government formerly—because of differences in regulatory politics and the more severe nature of many of the diseases that were the targets of older vaccines—had a heavier hand in fixing or negotiating low prices or demanding multiple suppliers for vaccines. Vaccines were therefore not necessarily big moneymakers, nor did they predictably give a large return on investment. In contrast, Gardasil's recombinant manufacture, along with changes in the regulatory environment, has made this vaccine much more like a highly profitable risk-reducing pharmaceutical product than the traditional biological vaccine, which was more highly valued as a public good but less profitable.

Gardasil's efficacy in reducing existing risk uncertainties

In terms of predictable economic and human costs, Gardasil's major impact is likely to be a reduction in the number of abnormal Pap smears, a direct result of the reduced incidence of infections from the vaccine-targeted HPV types. It has been estimated that less than

10 percent of the total economic costs associated with HPV infection ($4 billion annually) are direct medical costs of cervical cancer treatment.[27] Instead, the greater share of HPV's economic impact is due to the costs of screening and the work-up of the close to three million abnormal Pap smears in the United States yearly, especially the finding that has been termed atypical squamous cells of undetermined significance. If the vaccine ends up dramatically reducing the number of these abnormalities, as is expected, the cost savings might be immense. So would be the savings in hassle, fear, and wasted time of patients and doctors. This kind of efficacy has not been widely touted, certainly relative to avoiding cervical cancer, because it is essentially the reduction of iatrogenic costs associated with screening rather than improvements in the actual or objective health or well-being of individuals. This benefit would not accrue to populations where Pap screening is not currently done. But it is typical of a prominent type of efficacy within our risky medical paradigm—reducing the harm and costs of existing risk interventions.[28]

But the fact that there is something convoluted and self-referential about this benefit makes it no less real. It is a central and predictable consequence of our highly medicalized risk interventions. Looked at from this perspective, the initial construction and marketing of Gardasil as a drug against individual risk for Western markets is not an example of mistargeting but one that is right on target: Gardasil promises to reduce this noise in an existing expensive and wasteful risk-reducing system.

It is, of course, difficult to predict how much economic saving will actually occur. Gardasil may contribute to other trends that may increase medical costs. By increasing clinical and consumer interest in the HPV-cancer continuum, for example, Gardasil may lead to more HPV testing and its associated expense. There is already a direct-to-consumer advertising (DTCA) campaign aimed at increasing HPV testing. "Take the test not the risk" is the slogan of one such DTCA HPV test.[29]

Population goals one individual at a time

As mentioned earlier, vaccines have long held elements of individualized preventive treatment and population-level effects. But current vaccines are being researched, produced, and marketed in Western societies and medical systems in which risk identification and intervention at the level of the individual consumer have become central. So it is not surprising that mass immunization can strongly resemble mass-marketed risk-reducing products and procedures. In effect, vaccines, by means other than herd immunity or other contextual means, are being promoted as a one-person-at-a-time ("One Less") population-level intervention.

This scaling up of individual treatment to accomplish population health goals has become widespread. It is partly a response to criticism of the "high-risk" prevention strategy offered by proponents of population-level interventions. While high-risk prevention strategies can be meaningful and efficacious for the individual screened and treated, they often have only minimal relevance to the population because only the high-risk tail of the population distribution is impacted.[30] In contrast, population strategies aim to move the mean of the entire distribution "to the left." A population strategy for preventing heart disease might include changes in national food policy and zoning regulations that influence the entire population rather than screening and then treating individuals with high blood pressure and lipid levels. One retort to the criticism of high-risk prevention strategies has been to advocate for the mass use of preventive interventions that hitherto were used only for selected "high-risk" individuals. This is the last stop of the logic of risk intervention, made possible by high demand for risk reduction *and* population impact and permitted by the presumed safety and acceptable cost of some interventions.

This new paradigm in disease prevention has emerged following different paths. One path, the one followed by coronary heart disease prevention through the identification and treatment of individuals with high blood pressure, has been the gradual reformulation of the meaning of risk categories and their extension to huge swaths of the population. First, medicines were developed to treat hypertensive crises, then asymptomatic hypertension above a certain threshold was identified as a risk factor to be screened and treated, then this threshold was gradually lowered, and finally a new disorder, pre-hypertension—being at high risk for hypertension—was defined and promoted in such a way that a very large segment of the population could be labeled and treated.

The other path, today still more hypothetical than actual, is to put nearly everyone in the population on a hypertensive medication. Serious proposals for giving everyone a polypill—a concoction of low doses of safe, cheap, and efficacious medicines hitherto used to lower blood pressure, lipid levels, thrombus formation (aspirin), and hyperglycemic states—aim to move the population mean "leftward" one patient at a time.[31] Mass marketing of vaccines to individual consumers to become "One Less" cancer statistic shares many features with this brave new world of individual-by-individual population-level intervention.

Implications

It is possible that when vaccines are co-constructed as proprietary drugs against individual risk, they are in danger of losing their appeal as public goods. The proprietary character potentially undermines the belief that taking the vaccine is a civic responsibility rather than a consumer choice. As such, it may be a much harder sell to require them as part of school entry requirements or even to convince the public to voluntarily comply. Elements of this scenario already occurred with the recent failure of the Lyme disease vaccine (next chapter). Backlash has become routine in response to medications that have been advertised directly to consumers and for which demand has been manipulated in other heavy-handed ways. Witness the severe public outcry against Merck's funding of women legislators around the country and the backlash against the Texas governor—whose aide was formerly a Merck lobbyist—who attempted to mandate Gardasil as a vaccine required for school entry. Fueling this backlash is the apparent hypocrisy of the joint construction: dressing the vaccine as a public good but selling it and profiting by it as a consumer product.[32]

Many people have worried that Gardasil will be too expensive to be used in developing countries, where the burden of cervical cancer is greatest.[33] The high cost is one manifestation of a product conceived of and developed for the individual consumer who can afford it rather than the populations who most need it. This is perhaps the latest installment in a long history of the way different aspects of the economic and structural realities of American medical practice have interfered

6

Lyme disease vaccines: A cautionary tale for risk intervention

In George Bernard Shaw's play *The Philanderer*, Dr. Paramour reads with dismay a report in the *British Medical Journal* that proves that the disease that bears his name is nonexistent.[1] His patient with the hitherto-real Paramour's disease, sitting nearby, feels liberated and is annoyed by Paramour's despondency. Shaw's caricature of late nineteenth-century medical pretensions elicited laughs when I saw the play in 1982, but I wonder if it would today, when patients often cling more tightly to controversial medical diagnoses than their doctors.

One such prominent contemporary controversy is over the diagnosis and treatment of Lyme disease (LD). In many ways, LD is an unlikely battleground. It is an old-fashioned "new" disease. In the late 1970s and early 1980s, entomologists and clinical researchers rapidly identified the tick vector and causative bacteria, the spirochete *Borrelia burgdorferi* (named after its discoverer, Willy Burgdorfer). Diagnostic tests were developed and antibiotics were believed to be effective. These rapid developments might have led to a reassuring narrative about scientific ingenuity and medical efficacy. But events turned out differently. Nearly every aspect of the diagnosis, treatment, and prevention of LD has been fiercely contested.

What is Lyme disease? Who gets to decide? The major issue since LD was named and "discovered" has been the legitimacy and reality of *chronic* Lyme disease.[2] For many people in the LD lay advocacy community, LD is protean in its manifestations, often misdiagnosed

and underdiagnosed, and capable of causing months and years of de-
bilitating pain, fatigue, and anguish. From this heterodox perspective, which has become a formidable opposition to LD orthodoxy,
the chronic form of Lyme disease requires long-term, often-repeated
courses of antibiotics. In contrast, the orthodox position held by most
scientific experts is that LD is typically a straightforward acute infectious disease, readily diagnosed on the basis of rash and other clinical findings, with a supporting role played by laboratory tests, and
treatable by short courses of oral antibiotics. Late symptoms and syndromes can occur (rarely), but there is no need for repeated course
of intravenous antibiotics. Stricker, Lautin, and Burrascano called the
controversies over the definition, diagnostic criteria, and treatment of
LD the *Lyme wars* and noted that "suffering patients seek out 'Lyme-
literate' providers because the 'academic' researchers have failed
them."[3]

The stakes in these controversies are high. The question of whether
a protean condition called chronic Lyme disease with many different
subjective and objective manifestations exists and should be treated
with one or more courses of intravenous antibiotics remains the central issue. In a prominent consensus statement endorsed by the Infectious Disease Society of America (IDSA) in 2006, orthodox physicians stated that the evidence supported only three narrowly defined
late manifestations of LD (Lyme arthritis, late neurological LD, and a
rare skin condition called acrodermatitis chronica atrophicans), each
characterized by objective diagnostic criteria in addition to subjective
complaints, and for which there were only limited indications for a
single course of intravenous antibiotics.[4] Not only was this interpretation of the evidence contested by the heterodox community, but the
IDSA was subsequently subjected to antitrust action by the Connecticut attorney general.[5]

The heterodox position on LD could be said to have started with its
first patient, Polly Murray, who believed that investigators and doctors whom she respected and collaborated with were "playing down
the severity of the illness" as well as focusing too narrowly on arthritis
and other objective complaints.[6] Local support groups were started in
the 1980s to provide patient and physician education, practical support for patients, and fund-raising (Murray was involved in each of
these activities), often in tandem with the Arthritis Foundation, but

were shortly superseded by national and local groups that positioned themselves in opposition to the leading Lyme disease physicians and scientists and their view of the disease. The most prominent among these opposition groups are the Lyme Disease Foundation, the Lyme Disease Association, and, more recently, the International Lyme and Associated Diseases Society. But the networks of heterodox patients and their families and fellow-traveling physicians are close-knit, largely independent of organizations, held together by informal meetings and collaborations, and aided by the Internet.[7]

Twenty years after LD made its appearance in the United States, controversy erupted over the efficacy and safety of new LD vaccines. At first glance, these vaccines, like LD itself, might have followed an uncontroversial script. Two pharmaceutical companies, in concert with leading scientists and clinicians, developed similar vaccines based on a B. burgdorferi outer surface protein (OspA). Developing an effective vaccine faced steep challenges. In general, we do not have effective vaccines for infectious diseases such as malaria, which do not reliably produce immunity against subsequent disease. People can get LD multiple times. Ingeniously, the LD vaccines worked by blocking transmission of B. burgdorferi from the tick vector to the human host. Vaccine-induced OspA antibodies in the tick's human blood meal neutralize B. burgdorferi within the tick itself before it is transmitted to humans.

After animal and laboratory studies, two different vaccines based on the OspA antigen were tested in human populations and found to be effective and safe in premarketing clinical trials. Yet one of these vaccines was never submitted for FDA approval, and the other was withdrawn from the market by the manufacturer after only a few years of use. Why did these promising vaccines fail? What does their failure tell us about risk and efficacy in modern U.S. medicine and society?

What happened?

In the 1990s, SmithKline Beecham (SKB) and Connaught Laboratories independently conducted extensive laboratory and animal studies of OspA vaccines and then launched highly publicized phase III clinical trials involving large numbers of volunteers and clinical sites.[8] The main difference between the two vaccines was that SKB's LYMErix contained an aluminum adjuvant (often used to boost immunity) while Connaught's ImuLyme did not (which theoretically might lead to fewer side effects). In order to maximize the signal-to-noise ratio in a disease whose diagnostic criteria and boundaries had long been subject to intense controversy, both trials used narrow, objective criteria for what would constitute a Lyme disease case in the study population. "Definite" Lyme disease was defined as the presence of erythema migrans (EM, the characteristic LD rash) or objective neurologic, musculoskeletal, or cardiovascular manifestations of LD, plus laboratory and/or tissue confirmation via biopsy of rash. Such criteria maximized the specificity of the diagnosis and minimized the possibility of mistakenly seeing no preventive effect of a vaccine when one existed, which might result if many wrong or questionable cases were counted as LD.

The results from the two trials suggested that both vaccines were safe and effective. Numbers of nontrivial adverse reactions were similar in controls and subjects. Subjects who received the full three doses had at least a 75 percent reduction in definite LD compared with controls, and in the second year of the LYMErix trial (the only one to study this question), there were no cases of asymptomatic infection (defined by laboratory evidence of infection without symptoms) in the treated group. The absence of asymptomatic seropositives among the vaccinated could be understood as powerful evidence of vaccine efficacy because asymptomatic seropositive cases are ascertained only by objective measures, unlike clinical diagnoses, which might be counted mistakenly on the basis of how trial subjects perceived and reported symptoms and sought medical care and differences in physicians' diagnostic practices.

The trials also produced a disturbing picture of the inaccuracy of clinical diagnosis. In both trials only a small fraction of initially suspected cases were confirmed as definite Lyme disease (in the 10 percent to 20 percent range), suggesting widespread overdiagnosis (or alternatively, that the diagnostic criteria were too narrow). Because these data were from the carefully observed conditions of a well-funded clinical trial, a much larger problem certainly existed in everyday clinical practice. At the same time, a high percentage (30 percent) of cases confirmed by biopsy of skin rashes in the LYMErix trial were not accompanied by positive serology, suggesting that underdiagnosis was also present in the world outside trials, especially when clinicians depend on serology, for example, in cases presenting without the characteristic rash or after rash was gone.

The FDA licensed LYMErix in 1998 after a hedged recommendation for approval by its Vaccines and Related Biological Products Advisory Committee (VRBPAC). The committee's chair, Patricia Ferrieri, noted that "it's rare that a vaccine be voted on with such ambivalence and a stack of provisos."[9] After the FDA's approval, recommendations for use in clinical practice were taken up by the highly influential Advisory Committee on Immunization Practices (ACIP) of the Centers for Disease Control and Prevention (CDC). Some ACIP members considered LYMErix to be a "yuppie vaccine," its "manufacturer-driven and consumer-driven" market limited to worried suburbanites who "will pay a lot of money for their Nikes and their Esprit and shop at L. L. Bean's [and] will have no consideration for cost effectiveness when they want a vaccine because they're going to travel to Cape Cod."[10]

ACIP members concerned with this "yuppie vaccine" steered the committee to a lukewarm "should consider" recommendation for people at high risk and a "may be considered" for others "exposed to tick-infested habitat but whose exposure is neither frequent nor prolonged."[11] ACIP member Paul Offit noted that it was highly unusual for such a lukewarm recommendation to be given to a vaccine approved by the FDA.[12] In addition to the small numbers of people who would unambiguously benefit, support for LYMErix among regulators and advisory boards was hedged because (1) the trials had excluded children, limiting the vaccine's use until the efficacy and safety for children was established; (2) boosters were probably going to be needed to keep a high enough concentration of antibodies in the tick meal to kill spirochetes; and (3) concern that vaccine's side effects might appear with longer follow-up (especially concerns about vaccine-induced arthritis, discussed later).

The Connaught vaccine was withdrawn even before licensing. Connaught's anticipated market edge for ImuLyme may have evaporated when the vaccine was not proven to be any safer than the SKB product in the efficacy trials.[13] Leonard Sigal, the lead investigator on the Connaught vaccine trial, believed that the manufacturer concluded that marketing and other costs would be greater than the low revenues expected from the sales.[14] Connaught's competition, SKB, also had superior resources and experience to market their vaccine in the United States. Stanley Plotkin, a prominent vaccine researcher and consultant to the pharmaceutical industry, believed that there were record keeping problems in the Connaught trial that would have made regulatory approval difficult.[15] Although not privy to Connaught's decision-making process or drivers, Loren Cooper, an SKB lawyer, offered that it was not uncommon for one vaccine company to look at the experience of others when making development decisions.[16] In this instance, Connaught may have anticipated that the controversy surrounding LYMErix would also impact its vaccine and presciently decided to "stop the bleeding" rather than pursue a vaccine unlikely to be commercially successful.

One early warning sign of these problems was the report that volunteers in the clinical trials were suing vaccine manufacturers for the harm they experienced.[17]

Many of the problems with low demand were predictable far in advance of the pharmaceutical companies' decisions to withdraw their products. In most parts of the U.S., the disease is rare; it can be successfully treated by antibiotics and is not deadly. Most experts believe that LD complications like arthritis, Bell's palsy (temporary yet scary facial nerve paralysis), heart block, and back pain are infrequent, respond to treatment, and, even if untreated, eventually resolve. Infection can be prevented by individual measures such as tick checks and protective clothing. To the degree that these measures are a burden, a vaccine could never totally supplant them because ticks carry other infectious diseases besides LD and vaccine efficacy is never 100 percent. Because there is no person-to-person LD transmission, even the most effective vaccine would offer no protection to the unvaccinated (i.e., no herd immunity). So it remains puzzling why Connaught invested so much in vaccine development and its successful phase III clinical trial only to withdraw the vaccine before FDA approval or, similarly, why SKB anticipated a much larger market. I will return to this puzzle later.

At the time of the FDA's licensing of LYMErix, there were only limited data on long-term vaccine safety and the duration of immunity. Since the rationale for a vaccine against a "mild" and easily treated disease affecting small populations in specific regions remained marginal, regulators and others had an understandably cautious wait-and-see attitude toward the vaccine's safety, mandating SKB to conduct postmarketing surveillance (SKB agreed to set up a novel HMO-based surveillance system). At the time of licensing, regulators and others were quite concerned that the vaccine might induce an autoimmune reaction that would result in arthritis and other complications resembling the late complications of Lyme disease (discussed in greater detail later). On the efficacy side, there was great interest in whether the vaccine might prevent the intermediate and long-term neurological, rheumatological, and other effects of the disease.

During the 1998 VRBPAC meeting, Dr. Thomas Fleming pressed Allen Steere, the discoverer of LD and the chief investigator of the LYMErix trial, and others for evidence that the vaccine prevented these feared chronic manifestations. Steere told the committee that there were virtually no chronic or systemic problems, only one case with trigeminal neuropathy and one with Lyme arthritis. Since these sequelae also were rare in the placebo group, a reasonable interpretation of the very low rate of chronic or systemic problems was that the trial led to the prompt diagnosis and treatment of LD cases and such treatment was very effective at warding off later problems. This incidental and seemingly noncontroversial finding was one of many that would later put the organizers of the LD vaccine trials on a collision course with some LD activists.

When the VRBPAC met again in 2001 to review the safety and efficacy of LYMErix after more than two years on the market, SKB officials continued to argue that the vaccine was safe.[18] There was no evidence of a pattern of serious side effects reported either from usual adverse event reporting or from the HMO surveillance program. Despite some evidence of a link between the vaccine and musculoskeletal problems, there was no evidence of autoimmune reactions or treatment-resistant Lyme arthritis. "In all those studies the nature and the frequency of the adverse events were similar to the pre-licensure clinical trial experience," concluded SKB researcher Dr. Clare Kahn.[19]

But many Lyme disease activists and others at the advisory board meeting already had turned against the vaccine in a major way and were not buying SKB's assurances about its safety. Vaccine recipients at the meeting claimed that their health had been severely and negatively impacted by the vaccine. "I'm not as knowledgeable as this distinguished panel of experts that I speak to today," asserted one lay witness. "But I know one thing with all of my being. It was LYMErix which somehow had this devastating effect on my seventeen-year-old child."[20]

Some advisory panel members were puzzled by the disconnect between the reassuring adverse event reporting and the surveillance data presented by the SKB officials and the passionate narratives of physical and mental anguish following vaccination. Benjamin Luft, a prominent LD researcher, noted a failure to deliver on an earlier, if implicit, promise that in return for very quick approval of a "personal choice" vaccine, surveillance data would be collected to resolve lingering doubts about safety. SKB had been given "a gift," Luft argued. "I'm disappointed today. Because I hear some information here and I hear some information there. And I don't hear good data. We really are sitting in a situation in a sea of just what we feel. Because no one is giving us data."[21]

One reason that data were scarce was that the vaccine was being used much less often than predicted, making it difficult for either the adverse event–reporting system or the HMO surveillance program to reliably identify vaccine problems. The low uptake also signaled that the vaccine was in (market) trouble.

In February 2002, SKB, citing poor sales, voluntarily discontinued the manufacture and distribution of LYMErix. Dear Doctor/Investigator letters were sent, and refunds given for returned vaccine vials. SKB promised to complete all clinical studies.

A related dog vaccine has been very successful.

Heterodox opposition to vaccine

The preexisting controversy over the definition, scope, and significance of chronic Lyme disease would ultimately shape every aspect of the controversy over the LD vaccine. In retrospect, the developers of the LD vaccine did not fully appreciate what was at stake in these controversies and how these stakes would affect the reception of the vaccine. SKB gave financial support to different LD advocacy groups in the 1990s, presumably expecting them to be allies in bringing an effective and safe vaccine to market. They indeed might have helped turn the great concern about LD in endemic areas into vaccine sales, but instead, many LD advocates and the groups representing them ultimately turned on the vaccine and vaccine makers. As Loren Cooper, counsel to SKB for much of the ensuing LD litigation, put it in retrospect, given the discord within the medical community and among LD advocates and support groups, "We stepped into a hornet nest."[22]

One example of SKB's early strategy was the testimony on behalf of SKB and LYMErix at the 1998 VRBPAC meeting given by Dr. Robert Schoen, a physician and LD researcher. Schoen stressed LD's seriousness, arguing that the disease was analogous to syphilis. The etiological spirochete can "lurk or secrete itself in certain areas of the body, perhaps the central nervous system or perhaps the joint spaces, only to reappear months or maybe years later in the form of late stages of illness, which are harder to diagnose and treat."[23] He went on to show pictures of a patient with Bell's palsy and describe a patient with heart block, both real but rare LD complications. SKB's message was clear—the chronic complications of LD were serious and difficult to diagnose and treat. Because this message was consonant with the heterodox view of LD, it was therefore understandable that SKB might have expected significant enthusiasm in the LD advocacy community for an effective vaccine.

Yet the vaccine's social and psychological efficacy—the work it does or might do for potential consumers besides blocking *B. burgdorferi* in the tick's midgut—turned out to be complex and contradictory. From SKB's perspective, the vaccine promised to restore a sense of control and reduce the fears of many people living in an LD-endemic area. This work was crucial to developing a market larger than the relatively small numbers of individuals at high risk for *B. burgdorferi* infection. And even those at high risk needed additional reasons to take the vaccine, given the concerns about its cost, side effects, boosters, and incomplete protection.

But there were a few too many missteps and misunderstandings. More than putting pressure on scientific authorities to be included in the investigator-initiated research, LD advocates focused on garnering support and attention for their alternative picture of the disease as chronic and protean and often requiring prolonged treatment. Everything else was secondary. As the prominent LD researcher Alan Barbour wrote in an op-ed about LD advocacy at the very onset of the

LD vaccine controversy, "Most of the lobbying has focused on what Lyme disease is rather than how to prevent it."[24] Also absent from the heterodox opposition to the LD vaccine was any overt linkage to the long tradition of antivaccination campaigns in the U.S. in any of its guises: libertarian, religious, homeopathic, antimedicalization, and the like.[25]

A contentious point about "what Lyme disease is"—whether it was easily treated with oral antibiotics—remained, only exacerbated by the investigators' belief that chronic symptoms did not develop in trial participants because cases were accurately diagnosed and received oral antibiotics early. Dr. Dixie Snider, an FDA advisory panel member, recalled that VRBPAC's earlier "rather benign" observation that most LD cases were treatable with antibiotics resulted in "thousands of letters from the public indicating that that wasn't true."[26] Such a statement and the related findings in the vaccine trials were perceived as a direct attack on a core heterodox position.

The gap between the orthodox and heterodox positions has been wide and consequential. From the orthodox vantage point, many LD advocates did not deserve a seat at the table. It was as if people who had biopsies for breast cancer and tested negative demanded a say in how breast cancer practices and policies were being developed. Some LD advocates believe their children or partners died from Lyme disease, while most experts are skeptical that LD is ever fatal. Members of both communities frequently acknowledge they have been living in different and oppositional worlds. "Your reporting system might do well in the beltway," one patient advocate complained at the postmarketing regulatory hearings. "But out where the ticks are, out in the hinterland, nobody knows about it, or they are not telling you."[27]

One lay advocacy organization SKB initially supported was the Lyme Disease Foundation. At the 1998 VRBPAC meeting that ultimately gave approval to the vaccine, Karen Vanderhoof-Forschner, the organization's president, offered passionate support for LYMErix. Similar in many ways to the SKB-sponsored clinician who addressed the meeting, Vanderhoof-Forschner argued that LD was a geographically widespread, underdiagnosed, chronic, devastating, and costly disease—and thus worthy of prevention by vaccination. But in 2001 she told the same advisory board that the vaccine "represents an imminent and substantial hazard to the public health and needs to be immediately recalled."[28] Why did she change her mind so quickly? LD advocates were not, of course, against preventing the disease per se but were against the way the vaccine might reinforce the idea that LD was an acute, unproblematic, clinical entity. For many in the heterodox community, the vaccine, the vaccine's scientific efficacy, and the narrow disease definition had become mutually reinforcing concepts. Once the vaccine's efficacy was established, there was a collateral implication that the narrow diagnostic criteria used to establish this efficacy "worked" as well. This type of stabilization of both the technology and its target is sometimes understood as "coproduction" in science and technology studies. The heterodox antipathy to the vaccine also might have followed from the potential impact of widespread vaccination to reduce the ability of people to claim they had LD. Although there was never any evidence of this motivation, it was clearly in the minds of LD vaccine supporters. David Weld, executive director of the American LD Foundation (perhaps the sole advocacy group that supported the orthodox position), in testimony at the 1998 ACIP meeting had wondered out loud if the vaccine "may be very beneficial in that it's going to reduce the incidence of a lot of people claiming to have Lyme disease when they don't."[29]

While the efficacy trials, the adverse event reports, and the HMO surveillance system had not found evidence of the vaccine's dangers, the 2001 VRBPAC meetings heard a lot of testimony of individuals claiming serious harm. "What disturbs me is that in the SmithKline presentation there were 950 adverse events," chair Robert Daum noted.

> There was a nice presentation of that. And this afternoon we heard testimony from 20 individuals of twenty, of approximately twenty people who had very significant adverse events. And the disconnect for me is I'm hearing that, and I'm seeing that data, and I don't see any reflection of one to the other as if we were in two different universes.[30]

Not only were different types of evidence (statistics comparing the vaccinated and controls with the personal narratives) marshaled, but some heterodox advocates offered radically different interpretations of the same evidence. Rather than understanding the absence of asymptomatic seroconversion among the vaccinated as evidence of vaccine efficacy, some detractors offered a diametrically opposed interpretation: the vaccine caused people with prior or latent infection to become symptomatic with a LD-like disease—resulting in no one left to be asymptomatic. As one vaccine skeptic put it, the vaccine "is turning asymptomatic Lyme disease into symptomatic cases."[31] Kay Lyon, another vaccine skeptic, argued that asymptomatic infection was better understood as a "smoldering" infection and that the vaccine "might be a trigger that turns this smoldering infection on, converting it almost instantly into late stage disseminated Lyme disease." In support of the view that asymptomatic infection could later turn into serious disease, she noted that asymptomatic seroconverters, whom the research was designed to detect, had been treated with antibiotics by study investigators. Lyon continued: "this was, of course, the humane way to treat study participants. But it is absolutely not reflective of medical practice in the real world our children live in."[32] Again, LD advocates proved adept at using insiders' knowledge of how research and clinical care were conducted to score points for the heterodox position.

Some heterodox objections to the vaccine echoed a standard observation made by historians of technology and science: scientific practices and technologies often have built into them the choices, values, and interests of specific groups. Critics observed that the values and interests of LD experts and pharmaceutical companies shaped the design of vaccine and drug clinical trials, which in turn shaped beliefs about what was true about LD and everyday clinical practices. There was in effect great path dependency to some initial decisions and commitments made by scientists, clinicians, and regulators who shared the orthodox view.

Exhibit number one for this line of criticism was the relationship between the vaccine and diagnostic criteria for LD, long a battlefield in the Lyme wars. Many people in the heterodox community were incensed when in 1994, years before the launch of OspA vaccines, experts at a consensus group meeting in Dearborn, Michigan, sponsored by the CDC, removed from the diagnostic criteria a Western blot band associated with an antigen likely to be part of the LD vaccine. This band was removed so that the immunological tests would not be "fooled" by vaccination, that is, falsely diagnosing LD among the merely vaccinated. Some LD advocates objected that some infected people would be excluded from their "rightful" LD diagnosis because of these changed criteria. In effect, these would-be LD patients, now ineligible for the diagnosis, were sacrificed by the CDC experts in order to accommodate a vaccine of dubious value. One LD advocate observed that the changed laboratory criteria meant that it was now

> impossible for us to know which of our children are infected, and which are not. It is therefore impossible to gauge the true safety or efficiency of this vaccine, efficacy of this vaccine in this population … On the other hand in the world of SmithKline Beecham data we do find LYMErix, we have an experiment whose success is based, in part, on a set of criteria created to enable the success of the experiment.[33]

From the orthodox perspective, arguing that different bands on Western blots should be used to define LD was an intrusion into matters best left to the experts. And observing that diagnostic criteria were changed to minimize the chance that vaccinated people might later be falsely diagnosed with Lyme disease was sensible and unexceptional clinical policy.

Heterodox critics pointed out that the surveillance systems used to identify vaccine complications were imperfect and rigged to underreport problems. Reports of adverse reactions depend entirely on the willingness, energy, and competence of the physicians in practice. Side effects would not be reported if physicians believed they were not related to vaccine exposure. So recognizing adverse reactions was, in effect, a closed, circular system, in which preexisting biases shape reporting, which in turn reinforces these biases. No wonder there was underreporting of the vaccine's side effects. "When asked if they had reported this to the administering doctor, and if the doctor had reported the adverse event," lay advocate Pat Smith observed, "the usual response was that the doctor did not take the complaint seriously, or did not think that these symptoms were related."[34]

SKB had promised to make adverse event reporting more sensitive and objective by establishing a surveillance system based on electronic medical records of a large managed care system in New England. But vaccine use was much less than expected, making surveillance difficult. At the postmarketing regulatory hearings, some LD advocates heavily criticized this program, even though the low uptake that made this surveillance system a failure was partly due to activist opposition to the vaccine. They argued that postmarketing surveillance had made guinea pigs out of vaccine users. "We had no idea that there were unresolved safety issues requiring further study," one advocate observed about the licensed vaccine, "and that by taking this vaccine our family would unwittingly become subjects of an ongoing drug trial."[35]

The vaccine's immune danger

The case against the LD vaccine was different from what inspired opposition to other vaccines in recent decades. Higher than expected levels of Guillain-Barre syndrome had ended the 1976 swine flu immunization program; increased numbers of intussusceptions had led to the recall of an early rotavirus vaccine just around the time LYMErix was first being marketed; and the alleged link between MMR vaccine and autism have been a simmering controversy since the time of the LD vaccine controversy.[36] The main case against the vaccine was that it *caused* LD-like complications.

This concern about the vaccine has its origin in the belief that some late-stage complications of LD were caused by immune mechanisms rather than direct effects of the infection. In particular, LD experts have speculated that some LD-associated arthritis, particularly cases that are not responsive to antibiotics, is due to the body's immune attack on joints triggered by spirochete infection. Evidence for an autoimmune explanation of "treatment-resistant" LD-associated arthritis has included clinical similarities with rheumatoid arthritis, long understood as an autoimmune process, and the failure to find spirochetes in the affected joints.

It is a small step from belief in an autoimmune mechanism for LD-related arthritis to concerns that the LD vaccine could induce autoimmunity. What if the antigens used in the vaccine were the same spirochete bits that cause autoimmunity following natural infection? Moreover, the heterodox community frequently cited autoimmunity as the mediating mechanism for the chronic fatigue, pain, and other signs and symptoms that were prominent—and most contested and feared—in the alternative LD construction. If the vaccine itself caused a syndrome that was the same as or similar to chronic Lyme disease, then these "side effects" constituted evidence in support of the alternative disease definition. And if the vaccine did not cause these symptoms, then the heterodox position, to which putative autoimmune mechanisms were central, could be undermined.

These uncertain and contested beliefs about autoimmunity were the fertile soil from which opposition to the vaccine arose. Central to the case against the vaccine was the considerable scientific speculation in the years just before the vaccine's introduction that OspA was itself was the culprit antigen that triggered treatment-resistant LD arthritis via molecular mimicry. Allen Steere, who is credited with discovering LD in the 1970s, did much of this research. He had suggested a possible connection between individuals who express HLA DR4 antigen (HLA antigens play crucial roles in distinguishing self from nonself and are frequently evoked to explain who develops autoimmunity), exposure to OspA, and subsequent treatment-resistant arthritis. There was some evidence that the OspA protein was similar to a human protein named LFA-1, which may play a role in autoimmune arthritis.[37]

To some observers, Steere's role in advancing and legitimating these concerns was paradoxical. After all, he helped develop the vaccine and also led the LYMErix clinical trial while simultaneously championing a theory that suggested that the vaccine might be dangerous. Why would you develop and study a vaccine against Lyme disease that you had serious reason to believe might cause some of its late manifestations?[38] According to a *New York Times* profile, Steere "has his doubts about the safety of the vaccine."[39] But a less contradictory interpretation of Steere's actions was that he believed that OspA's role in autoimmunity was still an unproven hypothesis and the potential benefits of the vaccine were likely to trump any harm done by treatment-resistant arthritis. Pursuing the mechanism of LD-related arthritis and the efficacy and safety of the vaccine were both valid and important scientific efforts. In any event, the OspA molecular mimicry hypothesis subsequently fell out of favor, and neither clinical trial produced evidence of vaccine-induced arthritis.

Yet the theoretical concern about the vaccine causing LD-like damage persisted as the basis for vaccine opposition. A well-publicized suit against the vaccine, settled by SKB in 2003, was based on the manufacturer's liability and responsibility to the class of people *at risk for* an autoimmune reaction.⁴⁰ Promises were made about the language of a future package insert if the vaccine was ever reintroduced and attorney fees (but no patient damages) were paid.⁴¹

Because the LYMErix trial did not result in greater numbers of arthritis cases, treatment sensitive or resistant, SKB did not include any warnings about autoimmunity in the LYMErix package insert. What seemed logical to the orthodox camp was evidence of cover-up or hubris to the other side. At the 2001 VRBPAC meeting, advocate Jenny Marra testified that

> SmithKline was so concerned with this issue [possible autoimmunity] that they had study participants sign a paper indicating the theoretical possibility existed that vaccine might cause arthritis in certain genetically susceptible individuals. Yet SmithKline did not include this information in the product labeling, or inform the health care providers of this concern. Had I known this, I personally would not have taken the vaccine.⁴²

Autoimmunity has long been a fertile imagined space for etiological thinking about chronic diseases whose causes are unclear and that are characterized by exacerbations and remissions. Many of the psychosomatic diseases of midcentury (asthma, hay fever, and ulcerative colitis) were in subsequent decades reframed as autoimmune diseases.⁴³ While much of this was built on real and important new understandings of immunity, it was also the case that one appealing, intuitive, and flexible overriding causal scheme—psychosomatics— was replaced by another, autoimmunity.⁴⁴

The immune concerns about the LD vaccine have some parallels with drugs such as Tamoxifen and Finasteride, which have been tested and sometimes used to prevent breast and prostate cancer, respectively.⁴⁵ Despite some evidence of their scientific efficacy for prevention and regulatory approval, these drugs—when used as preventatives—have been market failures. In contrast, the screening tests for these cancers, mammography and PSA tests, are widely used despite controversy over their efficacy, overdiagnosis, and iatrogenic harm. One explanation is that these drugs, unlike screening tests, evoke different fears because of their direct effects on the body. Tamoxifen, for example, can cause uterine cancer and immediately produces menopause-like symptoms in many women.

Like Tamoxifen and Finasteride, the LD vaccines may be feared because of their putative direct effects on the body. In the case of the cancer preventatives, the comparison with the enthusiasm for screening is telling because the indirect effects of screening—overtreatment resulting from overdiagnosis—may be as consequential[46] but, I surmise, are feared less because their negative health impact is less direct.[47] The point is that social and psychological effects of practices and products, as much as or more than their scientific efficacy, often play a determining role in their actual use or rejection. Consumers worry that these preventives directly impact the body in unknown and uncertain ways, in one case towards cancer itself, and in the other toward murky immune problems. In each case, a preventive drug was marketed as reducing risk and controlling uncertainty/fear and yet has the potential to add risk and raise fears. As a result, many risk-reducing drugs and vaccines are unstable consumer products.

A personalized product?

At the postmarketing regulatory hearings, Dr. Richard Platt referred to LYMErix as a "personal choice vaccine."[48] At these same hearings, consumer activist Sidney Wolfe recalled an earlier IOM report that

> placed this whole idea in what they call their less favorable category, the lowest ranking in priorities of vaccine development, just because of the fact that A, the vaccine is not extraordinarily effective; B, it is not preventing a life threatening disease; and C for most people a successful antibacterial intervention can occur not when you have a tick, but when you have some clinical symptoms that are suggestive of actually beginning to have Lyme disease.[49]

Not everyone agreed that these characteristics of the vaccine and LD meant that the vaccine was optional and should receive less support or tighter regulation than most other vaccines. At the initial ACIP review in 1998, committee member Stanley Plotkin argued that a safe and effective vaccine with a limited market should nevertheless get a strong recommendation from policy makers. The issue of whether to actually use a highly recommended vaccine should remain with the individual. The LD vaccine, argued Plotkin, was

> the first of many . . . One is going to have to permit the individual to make some choices about whether a reduction from two in one thousand to one in one thousand is significant for that person. So I would urge the Committee to distinguish in this type of vaccine between public health issues and individual issues.[50]

In this new world of personal choice, vaccine manufacturers were motivated to persuade potential consumers. In the case of LD vaccines, consumers could be sold freedom from LD fears and the moral satisfaction following proper self-care for themselves and their family. So to succeed in the marketplace, vaccine makers would need to raise awareness of the risk of LD and also of the benefits of the vaccine.

After the FDA approved LYMErix, SKB launched one of the very first large direct-to-consumer advertising (DTCA) campaigns. "I never thought I was a target for Lyme disease . . . until I found out you can get it in your local park, in your own back yard, or even mowing the lawn," was the voice-over in one television advertisement.[51] A print ad from the same period pictured a woman who offered the following advice: "I got Lyme disease last spring and I'm being treated for serious health problems. I couldn't prevent it then, but now *you* could."[52] The campaign aimed to increase awareness of Lyme disease risk and communicate a sense of urgency about taking the vaccine.[53]

The DTCA campaign resembled the aggressive one Merck would use to promote its HPV vaccine, Gardasil, a decade later.[54] In both cases, the vaccine manufacturers promoted their vaccines as consumer choices, raising awareness and fear of the target disease and promising relief not only from the target condition (a benefit that would accrue to only a small segment of the population) but also from the anxiety, loss of control, and fear associated with being at risk for the disease. In both cases, vaccine manufacturers attempted to win over consumers by initially funding lay groups they believed could influence the vaccine's market success. In the case of Gardasil, Merck also took aim at state legislators who might vote to include Gardasil among the vaccines mandated for school entry.

Given the great degree of concern already present in some communities about LD, SKB had reason to believe that it had developed an economically successful vaccine. A prominent LD investigator speculated in 1999 that "one group who will demand it are people who fear Lyme disease with no real cause."[55] The vaccine's efficacy and safety in clinical trials only reinforced this promise. But the vaccine's social and psychological efficacy was quickly undermined by individual stories of harm related to the vaccine's putative immune dangers.[56]

Conclusions

Many informed observers of LD vaccine developments have offered explanations for why the LD vaccines failed. Allen Steere stated that "the withdrawal of the SKB vaccine . . . represents the most painful event in our Lyme disease history" and concluded that "the vaccine was really withdrawn because of fear and lawsuits, not because of scientific findings."[57] While there is a consensus among vaccine supporters that "scientific findings" had little to do with the vaccines' downfall, there is little agreement about which nonscientific factors were at work.

Many people have observed that there turned out to be not enough demand for the vaccine to be commercially viable. But almost all the factors related to either LD (e.g., it was treatable, nondeadly, and preventable by other means) or the vaccines (potential for inducing autoimmunity, need for boosters) that might have led to low demand were known prior to extensive investments in clinical trials, regulatory review, and initial marketing. So these disease and vaccine characteristics are better understood as supporting players, while the more fundamental causes are the more contingent and unanticipated actions that occurred in the brief period after clinical trials were finished and before LYMErix was withdrawn from the market. These actions tipped the balance toward the vaccines' demise. Specifically, we need to understand (1) the origins of the intense heterodox opposition to the LD vaccine and the weak orthodox support for the vaccines once challenged and (2) why the efficacy of a "personalized vaccine" was inherently vulnerable to this opposition.

Contingent events external to the LD controversy also influenced the market failure of LD vaccines—especially the controversies surrounding the RotaShield and MMR vaccines mentioned earlier—but I want to focus my analysis on the actors and actions within the developments concerning LD. Other ancillary influences include the theory offered by Sigal that the advocacy community turned against the vaccine when SKB withdrew its financial support and also the claim made by both Offit and Plotkin that the weak recommendations of the FDA and CDC/ACIP physicians' lack of enthusiasm for the vaccine.[58] The vaccine's supporters have blamed LD advocates for undermining the vaccine with nonscientific claims of its dangers, and SKB's vigorous DTCA promotion of LYMErix may have led to backlash and distrust.[59]

Heterodox groups came to believe that the vaccines' efficacy supported the orthodox definition of LD and did what they could to undermine the vaccines. These beliefs and actions were neither inevitable nor strictly determined by the clinical and biological characteristics of the disease or the vaccines. Early on in the vaccine story, major LD advocacy groups supported the vaccine. There was a great deal of enthusiasm in affected communities, as reflected in easy recruitment for vaccine trials and early lay criticism of the lack of medical interest in preventing LD. Speaking at the 2001 VRBPAC meeting, Dr. Dixie Snider recalled the very different atmosphere at the 1998 meeting, during which lay advocates told clinicians and scientists that they were insensitive to the needs of the communities who wanted the vaccine. But shortly after the launch of LYMErix, many people in the LD activist community began to understand that the vaccine's scientific efficacy stabilized the vaccine's target: the orthodox view of LD that they so bitterly opposed. Reinforcing these connections were lay activists' opposition to the LD experts and drug companies promoting the vaccine (my enemy's friend is my enemy), the narrow case definition used in the trials (if the vaccine worked, then so did the case definition), and the construction of the vaccine's immune dangers in ways that reinforced the heterodox position (severe side effects attributed to the vaccine proved the protean immune consequences of "natural" LD).

From the orthodox perspective, an effective prevention tool, the product of determined and creative laboratory and clinical science, was withdrawn because LD activists contaminated its potential market by spreading fear and confusion. But why was this lay opposition so effective at weakening the demand for these products? Labels like "yuppie vaccine" and "personalized vaccine," cited by medical experts in regulatory hearings, point to why the LD vaccines were extremely sensitive to efforts to paint them as dangerous. The social and psychological efficacy of risk-reducing products and practices is to provide safety, reassurance, fear reduction, and control of uncertainty. This efficacy was easily unraveled by LD advocates' promotion of the vaccines' putative immune dangers.

The LD vaccine controversy resembles the recent HPV vaccine controversy, explored in the previous chapter, in which societal wariness regarding another marginally effective, highly profitable risk-reducing product played a large part. The HPV vaccines have been resisted by groups suspicious of big pharmaceutical companies, some skeptical evidence-based medicine adherents, "abstinence only" supporters, and others. Unlike the LD controversy, there has not been a concerted attempt to link the HPV vaccine to a specific, if theoretical, safety risk. My analysis implies that such a risk might be the nidus in which a lot of other oppositional positions might form. In this sense, the LD vaccine controversy has more parallels to the recent controversy over Vioxx, a product whose market niche was to reduce risk (of gastrointestinal complications associated with other nonsteroidal anti-inflammatory drugs) but which was undone by evidence that the same product imposed a small but real risk of increased cardiovascular disease.

Risk-reducing products are especially vulnerable to actions that raise fear and damage trust and thus undermine the social efficacy of the product. LD activists were able to pollute the positive social and psychological efficacy by a small dose of personal anecdotes and theoretical concerns. This class of practices and products necessarily lives and dies by an "easy come, easy go" rule discussed in chapter 3—things that are easily and successfully promoted as relieving fear and reducing uncertainty can be just as readily undermined if they are shown—or believed—to be dangerous and risky.

The relatively weak and hedged support for the vaccine by members of both the VRBPAC and the ACIP also followed from the vaccines' identity as a risk-reducing product. While reducing fear, providing reassurance, and controlling uncertainty are valid consumer needs, medical experts were skeptical that they balanced out even a small health risk. Moreover, policy makers were concerned that "yuppie" or "personalized" vaccines, even if safe, might dilute trust in the entire vaccine enterprise by their marginal health impacts (see Sidney Wolfe's testimony).

LD activists asked whether scientific and clinical developments were "good or bad for the heterodox position" usually answered "bad" and acted accordingly. Some clinicians and scientists lived in a complementary universe in which the vaccine might have contributed to a favorable end to the LD controversies by reducing the number of people who had, or could claim to have, LD.

These fixed positions reflect a very long controversy that is ultimately about who gets to decide how LD is defined and, as a result, who ultimately gets the diagnosis.[60] Policy makers, clinicians, and vaccine companies failed to understand the central heterodox position that *patients* get to decide diagnostic criteria. SKB initially funded advocacy organizations and its DTCA campaign bypassed doctors, but the support these advocates craved was for the heterodox definition of LD, not an awareness of LD or a vaccine that stabilized the orthodox viewpoint and was created by the experts they loathed. With the benefit of hindsight, it might have made more market sense for SKB to have enlisted the support of more physicians and to have avoided any involvement with heterodox LD advocacy organizations.

This very established controversy over chronic LD has not gone away. Not long after the LD vaccines were withdrawn, the next major battle in the Lyme wars was over attempts by the Connecticut attorney general to sue a major infectious disease organization for monopolistic practices related to its consensus criteria for diagnosing and treating LD. This mobilization of antitrust laws against the typical ways expert physicians make and communicate consensus recommendations dismayed most medical observers but was seen by many in the heterodox community as a counterbalance to the power of the medical establishment to set the entry criteria for a much-coveted diagnosis and to discipline "Lyme-literate" practitioners.

More biomedical acceptance of the legitimacy of patient suffering, whether or not it fits an accepted diagnostic scheme, and clinical management strategies that focus on symptoms rather than specific diagnoses might go some way in lessening the heat of this thirty-five-year-old controversy over the legitimacy of chronic LD. But because this controversy is so entrenched, these patient-centered approaches run against more dominant reductionist tendencies in clinical care and are unlikely to have much impact.

The LD vaccine controversy is unlike controversies surrounding AIDS and other diseases that have also had a very determined and often oppositional lay advocacy.[61] These controversies often center on the inclusion of patients, minority groups, and other stakeholders in the planning and execution of clinical trials and policy making.[62] But Lyme disease is not AIDS. Advocates and experts have often lived in entirely different universes in which basic assumptions and motivations are built on the negation of the other. There has often been almost a totally incommensurate view of the opposing group's actions. Arguably, inclusion should not be valorized in itself but for what it brings: fairness, accurate research sampling, different perspectives, and so forth. The attempt to include the orthodox and heterodox perspectives in consensus conferences and other research and policy making venues has, by any standard, failed. Perhaps it is time to name and act as if Lyme disease and chronic Lyme disease were separate entities that have very little to do with each other.

Even if there are no ready solutions to the LD controversies, it remains important to understand what was at stake in the rise and fall of the LD vaccines because American medical practice is increasingly constituted by many similar risk-oriented interventions. The LD vaccine narrative reconfirms that the success or failure of risk-reducing practices and products depends heavily on different sorts of trust. Biomedical interventions that promise risk reduction are different from others that relieve pain, take away symptoms, or reduce suffering. The consumer of a risk-reducing product or practice has to place much more trust in aggregate probabilities of benefit and harm because these practices or products have no felt impact. At the same time, consumers do generally expect a more immediate effect from risk-reducing interventions. These interventions are often designed and promoted as practices or products that promise to restore control, combat fears, and lessen uncertainty. But if these same interventions are later linked to even small probabilities of risk or harm, this social and psychological efficacy can be easily undermined, and the trust shattered. The rise and fall of the LD vaccines shows just how hard it is for this trust to be maintained and how easy it can dissipate. And a lack of trust can easily be generalized to other interventions. At the postmarketing hearings, consumer activist Sidney Wolfe testified that the problem with the LD vaccines was that they reduced the public's faith in other public health measures.[63] He compared the situation to the "the tragic lesson of the swine flu vaccine . . . when one sees a very questionable immunization campaign such as this going on, about the implication and the negative effect on public health generally and on vaccinations in specific."

Knowledge of the social and historical context within which the LD vaccines became market failures may be useful to policy makers, especially as the number of health risk–reducing interventions— preventive measures, screening tests, and treatments aimed at reducing the probability of recurrence or new manifestations—is growing. This history suggests that the evaluation of benefit and safety of risk-reducing practices and products, which increasingly dominate medical care, should proceed with more nuanced attention to the challenges posed by their social and psychological and not only by their scientific efficacy.

In many cases, evidence-based, quantitative evaluations of objective health benefits and risks of interventions will profit from simultaneous identification and evaluation of the expected and actual social and psychological work done by interventions as consumer products. Currently, the consideration of such factors is marginal and not explicit and is carried out in an ad hoc fashion. In the formation of LD vaccine policy, regulators and expert clinical opinion clearly had misgivings about what was sometimes referred to as the "yuppie vaccine." These misgivings were partly a matter of the limited objective health impact of any putatively effective vaccine, but they were also about diluting the moral and political consensus that has stood behind vaccines as public health measures, and the dangers to medical credibility of blurring appeals to public and individual health benefits with consumerist benefits. Policy makers were, and remain, at a loss for dealing with the kind of oppositional lay advocacy manifested in LD. Even the pharmaceutical companies acting as market actors seemed to have misunderstood, at least initially, what might be at stake in their new product. Responding to these challenges necessarily involves simultaneous critical appraisal of extant data about the objective dangers and benefits of interventions along with their anticipated social, political, and economic impacts.

7

Cancer survivorship: The entangled experience of risk and disease

A 35-year-old friend was diagnosed with colon cancer and quickly had surgery followed by chemotherapy. In the aftermath, my friend and her husband decided not to wait any longer to have children. This proved difficult. They had known that chemotherapy might lead to infertility and had harvested eggs prior to treatment. But repeated attempts at in vitro fertilization and implantation were unsuccessful. Although profoundly disappointed, my friends moved onto plan B, adoption. They then learned, to their great dismay, that some foreign adoption agencies believed that a person with a history of colon cancer was an inappropriate person to adopt a baby. From my friend's perspective, she had been victimized by cancer three times: by cancer itself, from the assault on her fertility from chemotherapy, and then indirectly, by placing her in a class of people unfit to be mothers.

In common American usage, my friend is a *cancer survivor* and her problems are exactly the kinds of issues that the growing *cancer survivorship* movement hopes to make visible and ameliorate. Cancer survivorship is increasingly characterized by effects, like my friend's problems starting a family, that are mediated by the biological effects of the disease and treatment as well as by medical, social, and bureaucratic actions and reactions that follow from what we know or think we know about these biological effects. Uncertainty surrounds all levels and the interactions among them. Did chemotherapy play a major or minor role in my friend's infertility? What is my friend's prognosis from cancer? How should these uncertainties impact the allocation decisions of adoption agencies?

Cancer survivors are a rapidly expanding class of people. For many people, cancer survivorship has also become a career, way of being, or stage in the life-course. However large the number of cancer survivors and medically and culturally important cancer survivorhood has become, these developments have not been inevitable social and medical responses to cancer. Many aspects of American cancer survivorhood are specific to late 20th- and early 21st-century U.S. medicine and society. Other advanced industrial societies have some parallel developments, but a large-scale cancer survivorhood movement involving clinicians, patients, and lay groups has reached its apogee in the U.S.

Even the use of the same term, *survivor,* to refer to either "outliving" a plane crash or the disease cancer seems to be an Anglo-American peculiarity. According to a special European report on cancer survivorship, "in some languages (e.g., German, Dutch), no word for 'survivor' exists except as in the case of the survivor of an accident or violent crime."[1]

How and why did the person with cancer become a cancer survivor? What does it mean to be cancer survivor in the U.S. today? I seek answers to these questions by considering how terms like *survivor, cancer survivor,* and *survivorhood* have been used in different contexts. I pay special attention to the way these terms have shaped and been shaped by the experience of being a cancer survivor in recent decades, especially how for many people the cancer survivor experience has become one of perpetual risk. I conclude by suggesting a few problematic implications of this late 20th- and early 21st-century framing of the American cancer experience.

Survivorship: A problematic term and concept

Cancer survivorship as a term and concept deviates from the more prototypical meanings of *survivor, surviving,* and *survivorship* in other contexts. The prototypical referent of *survivor* is someone who experiences a deadly event or experience and outlives it. The closest use of *cancer survivor* to this prototypical meaning is the person who is quickly diagnosed and treated and lives cancer-free afterwards. But even in this situation, cancer can become a chronic condition; evidence of outliving it is necessarily provisional (one can only be said to have outlived cancer after one has lived cancer-free and dies of something else), and cancer is something that happens within rather than to someone. Unlike survivors of car or plane crashes, the cancer patient's catastrophe often exists potentially and ambiguously in the future. Even after seemingly successful treatment, cancer may persist or recur.

Yet to speak of *surviving* cancer is sensible, i.e., consistent with its noncancer usage, because the acute, past, external, and potentially catastrophic event may be the diagnosis itself, which can immediately trigger a confrontation with one's mortality, fear and anxiety, and a host of difficult decisions and medical interventions. A frequent saying in the cancer survivorship literature is that "the day one is diagnosed with cancer is the day one becomes a cancer survivor."[2] Whether due to the success of treatment or psychological accommodation, the cancer patient can be understood to have survived the diagnosis.

In noncancer contexts, *survivors* are often understood to be not only lucky but also cagey and resourceful. This connotation is part of the cancer survivor's meaning as well. Often claims are made that a cancer patient's personality or psychological state explains why he or she beat cancer or successfully adapted to punishing treatment and frightening uncertainty. This heroic view of cancer survivorhood—along with the idea that cancer can be an opportunity for self-growth—may explain some of its widespread appeal and the ease with which people take on or are given this label.

The term *survivor* in noncancer contexts is also used to denote family members or others who continue to live after the death of a husband, father, etc. This is the first meaning given in the *Oxford English Dictionary*. In obituaries it is common to say "Mrs. Jones is survived by her husband and two children." In newspapers prior to the 1980s this older usage was almost always the one used when the words "cancer" and "survivor" were juxtaposed.[3] Something closer to our current usage may have emerged from actuarial practice. A 1953 *New York Times* article quoted an expert who used life insurance survival tables to determine whether one cancer prevents you from having another cancer. These data concerned the "the life expectancy of cancer survivors."[4] This usage in statistical and epidemiological practice emerged from studies of the mortality experience of a cohort of cancer patients followed through time. In each time interval a certain number of this cohort die—the remainder are *survivors*.[5]

This usage had little of the cultural or clinical significance of survivorhood that was to appear in the 1980s. Precursors to cancer survivorship as an object of lay agitation and mobilization did occur in some site-specific cancers, notably breast cancer. In the 1950s, Terese Lasser started an organization focused on helping women with breast cancer and subsequently published a book titled *Reach to Recovery* that went through many updates and editions and that was largely concerned with the aftereffects of radical mastectomy and breast cancer on marital relations and feminine identity and appearance.[6] Both Lasser's book and a contemporary newspaper account of her organization focused on the potential blows to female attractiveness to men caused by mutilating surgery (marriage and heterosexuality were the unquestioned ideals).[7] The term *cancer survivor*, however, was not used.

In current usage, *cancer survivor* is often extended to any and every one "touched by cancer." There are even explicit definitions that include family members, although this is rarely how the term is used.[8] The cancer survivor category includes all stages of disease irrespective of one chances of outliving cancer or degree of suffering, threat to one's existence, or experience with treatment. Everyone alive who has ever been diagnosed with cancer is a survivor. At the population level, the prevalence of cancer of any particular site-specific cancer has become equivalent to cancer survivorship.

Cancer prevalence and therefore cancer survivorship has grown very rapidly, from 3 million in 1971[9] to nearly 12 million in 2007.[10] This rapid increase is not primarily due to an increase in the numbers of individuals who have cancerous biological changes in their bodies and much greater effectiveness of treatment and prevention. Both of these changes would need to be true to be consistent with the largely unchanged or modestly decreased cancer mortality in recent decades. Instead, this rapid quadrupling in cancer prevalence, and thus survivorship, is mostly due to extensive and highly sensitive screening, more diagnostic testing, lowered thresholds for pathological diagnosis, and the creation of many new "early" and precancerous conditions.[11] In the medical and popular literature, this expansion has often been discussed as *overdiagnosis*.[12]

What one believes about the causes of this dramatic increase in cancer prevalence has direct effects on the meaning and significance of cancer survivorship. Why cast as a hero someone who has been diagnosed with a disease that is unlikely to cause any harm? Such a person might be better understood as a victim of a labeling error rather than a cunning or lucky evader of a catastrophe. It also seems inappropriate to lump someone who outlived a cancer which typically kills or who is symptomatic from active disease with people who have a very small probability of suffering some harm. But there is at least one reason to accept such lumping: in as much as survivorhood now evokes the *career* of a cancer patient, even the person overdiagnosed often has to live with diagnosis and its associated fears and work as much as someone with a high likelihood of recurrence and death. For one thing, overdiagnosis is confidently appreciated only at the aggregate or population level. At the individual level, things are typically much murkier. These individual uncertainties are permissive conditions for the rapid expansion of cancer survivorship and greater uniformity in the cancer survivor's experience.[13]

As mentioned earlier, survival in noncancer contexts is usually defined relative to a specific event. But cancer is a very heterogeneous category, more of a catch-all term for many different disease processes. It subsumes, for example, the many different site specific cancers. Cancer includes mesothelioma, a type of cancer which invariably and quickly leads to death, as well as many types of skin cancer, which almost never do. This heterogeneity is partly due to the very different biological processes put under the cancer label. It is also due to how we define cancer in relation to its natural history, the ways we screen and treat different cancers, and the efficacy of these interventions.

So to speak of 12 million American cancer survivors is to lump and mobilize many disparate clinical situations and individuals. Cancers whose prevalence and clinical course have been only marginally changed by modern medical interventions are lumped with cancers which have been transformed by how we find, identify, and name them.

And as the numbers of cancer survivors has grown, people whose situation used to be prototypical of the cancer experience now poorly fit the category. Take lung cancer, a disease which has not been effectively treated or medically prevented. Few people are cured, revealed by the fact that that lung cancer incidence and mortality are roughly equal.[14] Since the expectation for prolonged life after diagnosis is low, there is less use of the term *survivor* for people diagnosed with and treated for lung cancer. It is difficult in this situation to support those patient narratives that stress victory, heroism, hopefulness, wiliness, etc. It also hard to valorize patients whose cancer is often caused by a known, stigmatized, behavioral risk factor—smoking—that has over the last few decades been understood to be a danger to others. The current meaning of cancer survivorship follows from the disease's transformation by medical and social interventions into something less than a death sentence. Survivorship in its current optimistic and inclusive usage would have made very little sense in the nineteenth century, when the disease was thought to be uniformly progressive and deadly, with or without treatment.

Yet cancer survivorship makes no sense without knowledge or memory of the older meaning, since one would not speak of surviving a steady, slow chronic disease (e.g., we don't speak of diabetes survivors) or an infectious disease that continued subclinically in patients' bodies. Even a disease like AIDS, which shares many characteristics with cancer, is not typically understood as having survivors.[15] Perhaps we do not typically speak of an AIDS survivor because medical and lay persons know that in almost all cases, including people with no detectable viral load after retroviral therapy, the causative agent (HIV) remains in the body. In other words, cancer's older reality—a disease that uniformly and quickly led to death—permits the term *survivor* to be plausibly extended to people diagnosed with cancer and who live with some reasonable expectation of not dying from the disease. They are outliving cancer's older reality.

I do not want to overemphasize cancer's clinical features and historical transformation as the reason why cancer appears to be the only disease of which we routinely and consistently speak of survivors. Cancer survivorship, as a term and concept, has been widely used because it is performative, i.e., it does work that particular people and groups find useful. Researchers, clinicians, and different patient groups have used the term and extended its reach because there was something useful about uniting diverse individuals and biomedical phenomena into a unitary category based on the experience of a diagnosis. Its ambiguity is useful too. Cancer survivorship suggests something positive about both the labeled individual and his or her prognosis while not specifying what is positive in the experience or whether outliving cancer is a matter of psychology, lifestyle, medical intervention, labeling, or chance.

Some of these ambiguities have been analyzed and debated among members of the survivorship community with considerable sensitivity and passion. In one online discussion a woman with ductal carcinoma in situ (DCIS, a non- or preinvasive breast cancer that is often—and controversially—treated as or more aggressively than invasive cancer) had a bilateral mastectomy and was later told the good news that final pathology showed no invasive cancer in either breast (sometimes there is DCIS in one place and invasive cancer in another).[16] In the aftermath, she was still "suffering emotionally," one aspect of which was the potential ambiguity of her status as a cancer survivor. "Some of my friends say I am a breast cancer survivor," she wrote the group. "Yet I feel that I wasn't even close to that because there are so many women who have gone through SO much more than I. I feel as if I try to classify myself in that league—I'm cheating the women who have suffered through so much more. And yet—I'm still feeling the effects of having gone through something." This survivor's doubts about fitting the category are not—at least explicitly—a matter of the final pathology, but her degree of suffering.[17]

The resounding response from others in this forum was to support this woman's experience as genuine cancer survivorship. This support came from women with more advanced cancer and from other women with DCIS (interestingly, the signature line of many online postings is an abbreviated but detailed diagnosis and staging summary, e.g. "Diagnosis: 4/2010, IDC, 1cm, Stage I, Grade 3, 0/7 nodes, ER+/PR+, HER2"; this standardized, medical, and highly reductive identification is in some tension with the critical commentary in the website that celebrates the individuality of the cancer experience). One member of the forum wrote in reply that "your loss and your surgeries are just as profound as anyone of us who may have had a more advanced stage of cancer," emphasizing that it was the emotions ("loss") and interventions that followed from the diagnosis, whether it be a risk state or advanced cancer, that made one a survivor.

Another respondent empathized with the feeling that DCIS might somehow make one less authentically a survivor. "I don't feel worthy of the BC survivor title because there are so many women that battle this beast every day, while I was able to dodge the bullet with surgery, although serious life altering surgery." Yet she immediately added, "I struggle with emotions every day, I have a hard time explaining what I have, why I did what I did, every day." In this and other responses, the psychological struggle to find meaning and combat fears and uncertainty were constitutive of the cancer survivor experience.

Other respondents added details about the nature of this psychological struggle. "You never completely get back that same comfort zone in regards to medical procedures and testing that you had before cancer. I know women that are 20 years past their diagnosis that still get on edge when they go for their screenings. We have post treatment issues that people who have never been diagnosed have no comprehension about, is that back and hip pain because I twisted and picked up my grandchild, or is it mets [metastasis]?" Another respondent made the centrality of the triggering diagnosis even more explicit: "I think surviving hearing the diagnosis of 'cancer,' with all the kettledrums and crashing cymbals that go along with it, is worthy of a 'Survivor' label." And another participant in this forum argued that "you're a breast cancer survivor because you are never able to go back to your comfort zone. All of us have been irrevocably changed and that is what makes us a survivor."[18]

From disease to risk: The end of "natural" history

One hundred years ago, the cancer experience in the U.S., which was not yet understood as survivorhood, began to undergo dramatic transformations. Prior to this time, cancer was generally treated haphazardly and with deep pessimism. Definitive diagnosis or treatment was rare. Although people were "touched by cancer," there was often no one single moment when the momentous diagnosis was given. Surgery, in the rare cases it was done, was not generally understood as curative.

Along with other developments, radical cancer surgery changed the experience of cancer in the early twentieth century. So-called "complete operations" for cancer in the breast, for example, helped catalyze a historically new stage of cancer in which women lived a "life at risk."[19] The promotion of extensive operations meant that surgeons had to agree on standardized criteria for the cancer diagnosis. Because radical surgery often removed any local trace of cancer, patient and medical attention after surgery was directed at signs and symptoms that might indicate an internal recurrence. Surgery's very extensiveness, along with the stirrings of public health campaigns that stressed the value of early cancer detection, encouraged patients to believe that finding recurrences "early" might prove beneficial. So during the postsurgical period, women surveyed their bodies for possible warning signs of cancer and sought surveillance examinations from physicians. Patients typically remained in a prolonged state of uncertainty and heightened risk since physicians had difficulty distinguishing cancer-related symptoms and signs from other processes.

Many physicians were also in no rush to definitively diagnose recurrences because they had little faith there was much to do about them. Physicians in the early twentieth century were developing new practices and technologies to deal with the inevitable return of cancer, including radium implants and external radiation, but these were "salvage" treatments, capable of producing temporary if dramatic reductions in tumors that did not ultimately cure patients. The new stage of postsurgery cancer, this "life at risk" experience, was thus more highly intervened-in and medicalized. Expectations of medical efficacy were raised by standardization, new practices and technology, and advances in medicine and surgery generally, but were not matched by significant changes in cancer mortality.

New attitudes, practices, and technologies had thus transformed the disease experience, at least for the minority of patients who underwent initial extensive cancer treatment. Afterwards, their lives were characterized by concern for the future, self and medical surveillance, and problematic decision making and doctor-patient negotiations, especially about these powerful "salvage" cancer treatments when problems resurfaced.[20]

By the latter half of the twentieth century, especially after the widespread use of chemotherapy for many cancers, the "life at risk" experience of this minority of cancer patients became much more common. Partly due to improved treatment for childhood leukemia and other cancers but mostly due to the rapid expansion of cancer prevalence due to early detection campaigns and changed diagnostic practices, more and more people were living longer after initial treatment and with some reasonable hope of a cancer-free life.

The cancer experience was also being transformed by the content of midcentury early detection campaigns. These campaigns aimed to reduce the stigma of cancer by stressing the heroic quality of sufferers and combated cancer fatalism and pessimism by stressing that cancer was not always deadly. These campaigns were not aimed at transforming the experience and self-understanding of those people diagnosed, but at the medical profession and the general public. But changes in the individual experience of cancer were collateral effects, especially as the cancer experience became much more of a mass phenomenon in the later decades.

These developments were the permissive conditions for the first talk of cancer survivorhood in the 1980s. In addition, the bewildering array of therapeutic and care innovations were making life with or after a cancer diagnosis a difficult terrain to navigate. Newspaper articles with titles like "Changing View of Cancer: Something to Live With" noted the odds of survival had become much greater at the same time treatments were becoming unending. There were constant physical and emotional reminders of the disease: symptoms, prosthesis, need for pills, and knowledge of future risks. There was a "new sense of mortality, added fear about the future and a sense of somehow being apart from those who never had cancer. Each new ache or pain, they say, brings with it a special terror that their cancer is growing or spreading."[21]

In the mid-1980s, organizations like the National Coalition of Cancer Survivorship appeared, and in 1996 the National Cancer Institute established an Office of Cancer Survivorship. In 1985, physician Fitzhugh Mullan wrote an influential *New England Journal of Medicine* essay, drawing from his personal experience with cancer and his own clinical observations, which argued for three *seasons* of survival. A life preoccupied with the aftershocks of a cancer diagnosis and initial treatment, *acute survival*, was followed by one full of watchful waiting and intense surveillance, *extended survival*. After some period cancer-free one could assume a cure, drop surveillance and treatment, and enter into a period of *permanent survival*.[22]

Mullan's *extended survival* roughly corresponded to the "life-at-risk" experience of early twentieth-century cancer patients after radical treatments. By the end of the twentieth century, this once-rare stage had become common. At the beginning of the twenty-first century, we are rapidly eliding the difference between Mullan's last two categories. Aspects of extended survival—different types of surveillance and concern—have become permanent features of the post-diagnosis experience. Knowledge about risks associated with ever having had cancer and expanding regimes of surveillance and secondary prevention have at the same time undermined Mullan's *permanent survival* stage.[23]

New types of knowledge and interventions have also undermined a linear, temporal stage-based cancer experience. Risk is no longer a state that precedes disease, but occurs anywhere along the cancer experience trajectory. It permeates the experience before, during, or after the cancer diagnosis. Perhaps the most common experience of survivorhood, being touched by cancer, is coping with risk. Risk insinuates itself into decisions about screening, surveillance, and lifestyle change. It is simplistic to think of survivorship as some late stage in the course of disease or that the cancer experience is tied to different stages of the natural history of cancer. In many ways, we have made obsolete—at the experiential level—the orderly, stage-after-stage, biology-driven natural history of cancer. One can be touched by cancer without or before a diagnosis and long after treatment or last evidence of active disease.

Cancer survivorship might begin prior to definitive diagnosis, when a man gets a telephone call from an estranged sister who tested positive for a Lynch syndrome (a familial cancer syndrome) gene, immediately presenting him with uncertainties and different testing and screening decisions. Cancer survivorship might characterize someone diagnosed with cancer but who has opted for no treatments. This not uncommon situation occurs when cancer is not treated initially because "watchful waiting" is a viable option, for example many men with good-prognosis prostate cancer. For some "early" cancers, the diagnostic biopsy may have removed cancer from the body—so the moment of diagnosis may also be the moment of apparent cure. Or, as in the case of lobular carcinoma in situ (LCIS), a breast "precancer," current medical opinion is that the tissue removed by biopsy is more a marker of increased risk of later cancer rather than itself being the physical precursor to later disease. At the other (later) end of cancer's natural history, there may be no point in an individual's cancer experience when surveillance or treatment is in the past. The cancer experience may be dominated by the management of risks associated with the cancer itself, advancing age, prior treatments, and physiological or other sources of individual variation.

The new survivorship thus often implies, in apparent contradiction, finality ("living beyond") and endlessness ("living with"). Cancer survivorhood corresponds to the reality that one always is "touched by cancer" even if one is seemingly cured after biopsy or initial treatment or "merely" at risk of disease on the basis of family history, genetics, environmental exposure, or lifestyle. The everyday meaning of surviving suggests that one has evaded a potential catastrophe and can now move on with his or her life, while for many cancer is never really in the past. Not only is it remembered, but it often becomes a kind of essential identity, a career devoted to dealing with the knowledge of risks and aftereffects. We thus speak of "survivorship" or "survivorhood."

Survivor's flexible and ambiguous meaning works to sustain these contradictory ideas, especially with regards to agency and responsibility. A survivor can be either a victim of external events or a wily individual in control of his or her destiny. Surviving can be understood as a meaning-giving opportunity or a stark confrontation with a meaning-extinguishing death. It can be an open invitation to medicalize more with standardized surveillance protocols or to find one's individual way. Survivors can be compliant with these routines or use the survivor umbrella as a way of organizing an oppositional activism.[24]

The new phenomenon of *previvorhood*—cancer survivorhood for people who are at risk of cancer but never actually diagnosed—is additional evidence of survivorhood's divorce from older models of cancer's natural history.[25] People who are at high risk of cancer, say because they have tested positive for a mutation of a gene that is highly associated with developing cancer, may elect for prophylactic surgery. Witness the dramatic rise in both prophylactic bilateral mastectomies for genetic and other risks and contralateral mastectomies in the unaffected breast of women with breast cancer. In the former case at least, women may never have been diagnosed with cancer, but because of risk states and punishing treatments they may understandably feel that they have survived something. Their lives can be quite similar to others who in a more direct way can be said to have survived cancer (chapter 2).

The "risky" work of being a survivor

Recent reviews of cancer survivorship and clinical guidelines suggest the multitude of risks posed to cancer survivors from the original cancer, surgery, radiation and chemotherapy.[26] As a result, survivors are often advised to make lifestyle and dietary changes, comply with surveillance tests, and take prophylactic medicines through the rest of their lives.

Cancer survivorship is often experienced in unpredictable and non-standard ways. Its clinical management is largely an experimental zone in which innovation and guesswork dominate. Despite the increasing rhetoric for evidence-based medicine and standardization, medical care for survivors is often characterized by improvisation.

A friend in his seventies was recently diagnosed with a good-prognosis prostate cancer following PSA screening and ultrasound-guided biopsies. After a few consultations and his own review of medical literature and internet sources, he decided to do "watchful waiting" rather than surgery or radiation. His urologist proposed to do frequent rectal exams, PSA and free PSA determinations, ultrasounds, and MRIs at different intervals over the next months and years. The use of these surveillance practices did not follow well-researched protocols. Instead, this urologist and others have largely improvised their own rules for how and when to be concerned with evidence of progression or be reassured or not by other results. My friend's urologist could not specify with much precision what results would trigger particular actions. There were too many potential variables in play. My friend's situation was simply too unique to compare to a corpus of extant clinical knowledge.

The centrality of idiosyncrasy along with the obliteration of a temporally ordered natural history of cancer discussed above represents a return in some ways to a much older *constitutional* way of understanding cancer and ill health in general. Cancer is a constitutional disease not because we have returned to thinking about it in nonspecific terms or as a disease "of the blood" with fluid hereditary and environmental determinants. Rather, cancer survivorship is built from a web of statistical knowledge with so much inherent randomness and variation that can be made sensible only in individual terms. Individuals differ in how cancer was diagnosed and treated as well as in their medical history, underlying health, and lifestyle. Along with variation in biological characteristics of tumors, these multiple determinants mean that individuals after diagnosis and initial treatment often have a unique and often difficult-to-predict health trajectory.

In general, medical research has been focused on initial cancer diagnosis and treatment. There have been few standardized approaches to determining prognosis or deciding on a course of surveillance and intervention for individuals who make different initial treatment decisions and have had different staging, clinical presentations, and underlying health, values, and experience. And even if there were more randomized clinical trials in this area, they would necessarily be structured to see whether one particular intervention is better than another, not to capture individual differences.

Being a cancer survivor often means dealing with uncertainty and incompleteness. The survival experience can be dominated by risks. Some interventions are appealing because of their potential to reduce or eliminate this risk state. Doctors explain that they offer surgery for good-prognosis prostate cancer because they believe most patients find the work and worry of intensive "watchful waiting" unbearable.[27] As explored in chapter 3, the efficacy of many surveillance routines and thresholds for intervention can best be understood in social and/ or psychological terms. Hope may be sustained, patients may worry less about being abandoned, and fear and uncertainty—the doctor's as well as the patient's—can be reduced.

As risk becomes embodied, dense with nodal points and decisions, filled with other medical routines, it becomes a state to be avoided and worthy of prevention itself. The interventions that define previvorship, for example prophylactic mastectomy, are often done to gain completeness, to return to a state of certainty, and to banish risk. In addition to previvorship interventions, we also have vaccines against risk states, such as the HPV vaccines (see chapter 5).

But many cancer screening and surveillance interventions do not so much banish risk as recalibrate it, leading to new uncertainties and incompleteness. Someone like my friend with good-prognosis prostate cancer who is watchfully waiting is likely to receive frequent blood tests, ultrasounds, physical exams, and biopsies. He may watch his apparent risk go up slightly, unsure whether this is a trend and if so, what it means. After a period of watchful waiting, many men and their physicians opt for radical surgery or radiation to put an end to the risk-dominated state of incompleteness.

This social efficacy of many cancer interventions, the reassertion of control over feelings of randomness, uncertainty, and foreboding and putting an end to the many negative and difficult aspects of survivorhood, is typically ignored in the formal evaluation and explicit medical debate about specific practices. Yet it helps explain why many cancer survivors and physicians crave or require more immediate, experienced, or witnessed kinds of evidence.[28] Regardless of whether results of surveillance directly suggest one course of action or another, patients and doctors are heartened by evidence of partial or complete remissions, clean scans, reduced levels of tumor markers, etc.

This evidence, however, is often fraught with ambiguity. In the middle of Paul Tsongas's aborted attempt to win the 1992 Democratic presidential nomination, a controversy erupted over whether he was at the time "free" of cancer. Tsongas claimed he was, having been diagnosed and intensely treated for non-Hodgkins lymphoma (NHL) many years earlier. But reports surfaced that six years before his presidential bid, Tsongas may have been told that there were still cancerous cells in his bone marrow. Was Tsongas lying about being cancer-free? Did he have enough of a clean-enough bill of health to be president? One way to read this complex story is that Tsongas and his physicians were complicit in some purposeful ambiguity about the significance of a "recurrence" of his NHL following a bone marrow transplant. Tsongas may have been told he was *in remission* and that the natural history of some forms of NHL is such that the presence of some cancerous cells was still compatible with a long life and dying from something else. Tsongas ultimately died of complications from cancer recurrence in 1997, but during the election controversy it was unclear, perhaps purposefully so, what his status as a cancer survivor actually meant, both in terms of his prognosis and whether he was honestly representing it.

Implications

As I suggested earlier, one reason the cancer survivor label has been so widely adopted is the implication that the survivor is resourceful, cagey, and even heroic. The attachment of a heroic moral valence to cancer survivorhood shares something with the use of the term *Holocaust survivors* to denote people who experienced and outlived Nazi extermination campaigns.[29] Psychiatrist and one time concentration camp prisoner Bruno Bettelheim's criticisms of some widely held popular beliefs about Holocaust survivors point to some limitations of valorizing cancer survivorhood.[30] Bettelheim questioned different aspects of the popular reception of the survivor experience. First, he felt people exaggerated the degree to which evasion of extermination depended on the actions or personality characteristics of the survivor, when so much was determined by external, often random, events outside his or her control. Second, to the degree there was any agency in literal survival, Bettelheim observed that survival under such extreme and brutal conditions involved a radical restructuring of one's assumptions and behavior.

Bettelheim used the global success and critical acclaim given to the dramatizations of the survival of Anne Frank and her family in wartime Holland to underscore this latter point. The Franks' perseverance with normal family life and their slow but inexorable retreat into smaller and smaller hiding spaces was the wrong strategy for literal survival. Dispersion of the family (think of the prescience of families who made the heart-wrenching decisions to put children into kindertransport prior to the outbreak of World War II), and other improvisations that might follow from recognition of radically changed circumstances characterized more successful adaptation. Bettelheim understood the tragedy of the Franks' persecution and the emotional appeal of Anne's diary and the dramatizations of the family's story, but he was dismayed that their survival strategy was widely appreciated as heroic. But in whatever strategy chosen, Bettelheim deplored the casual moral standing or opprobrium attached to people on the basis of their outcomes. Similar criticism might be leveled at—and help explain—the contemporary American construction of cancer survivorhood, which exaggerates the consequences of individual action and valorizes survival qua survival, persevering with normal life and routines.

Bettelheim also addressed the issue of cancer survivorship directly, suggesting that the intensity of cancer practices and deep faith in their efficacy served to distract patients from death anxiety. According to Bettelheim, death anxiety was formerly relieved or managed with religion, being replaced by a quasi-religious faith in scientific and technological progress. Distraction from death anxieties is of course understandable, but the evident downside was a religious-like, exaggerated commitment to and faith in the power of medical interventions.[31] More recently, Jain echoed and advanced Bettelheim's criticisms by arguing against a "politics that tries to disavow death (as the survivor politics does)" and called for another kind of politics that might account for "loss, grief, betrayal, and the connections between economic profits, disease, and death in a culture that is affronted by mortality."[32]

There are negative implications for another aspect of the modern American survivor concept and movement: the lumping of individuals with wildly different prognoses and cancer experiences into a unitary cancer survivor category and the massive growth in the number of people so labeled. While there are some upsides to such lumping — growth in the numbers of survivors has led to greater societal and medical attention and more funding for research and clinical initiatives — the downsides have received less attention; I want to highlight a few of them.

Both societal attention and (more importantly) resources are limited. The cycles of increased screening, diagnostic expansion, and growing disease-specific survivorhood have resulted in large self-interested coalitions of affected individuals across the wide spectrum of risk-to-disease experiences. These coalitions, along with clinicians and researchers focused on cancer X or Y, are able to influence funding and other policy decisions potentially incommensurate with the "objective" burden of disability and death from cancer X or Y.

The rapid growth from three million to twelve million cancer survivors over a few decades, mobilized for medical surveillance and individual action, has obvious implications for fund raising, shaping political priorities, and markets for medical interventions and consumer products. At the beginning of the cancer survivorship upswing, a newspaper advertisement by a hospital that stood to profit from cancer survivorship interventions proclaimed "We have cancer programs for people who don't have cancer,"[33] underscoring the unbounded, limitless market for cancer surveillance and prevention among the apparently unaffected. Another advertisement promoted a talk titled "Surviving Cancer: A Whole New World" in order "to honor and celebrate more than 8,000,000 cancer survivors nationwide," featuring an author of a book titled *50 Essential Things to Do When the Doctor Says It's Cancer.*[34] In the time since these advertisements, the number of survivors and things to do have greatly increased—as have the number of hospitals and other market actors that stand to profit from this expansion.

At the individual level, the growth and meaning of cancer survivorship have sometimes obscured the experience of people with rapidly growing and difficult-to-treat cancer. Although "touched by cancer," many of these people have an uneasy fit within the survivor class. "You can see why patients with metastatic disease," an oncologist recently observed, "may feel invisible within the advocacy community."[35] And it is not only a matter of people with advanced disease being much more of a minority within the ever-increasing numbers of people with a good prognosis, previvors, overdiagnosed individuals, and people at risk. It is also a matter of outlook. Surviving implies victory and people with advancing cancer cannot claim to be vanquishing the disease. If the survivor is understood as a fighter, resourceful, wily, like a fox, it is all too easy to equate disease progression with failure. This equation ironically encourages the stigma and invisibility of the cancer experience that modern cancer survivorship was meant to combat.

There has been some understandable pushback from those who have observed that the general rhetoric surrounding cancer survivors is relentlessly optimistic and obscures and excludes the experience of people who are not outliving cancer. In a 2011 *New York Times* article, Elizabeth Edwards's discussion of her own cancer as incurable (she was to soon die of it) was depicted as courageous and honest while her philandering husband and ex–vice presidential candidate John's depiction of cancer as a chronic disease was held up as obfuscating and evasive.[36]

As previously discussed, the terms *cancer survivor* and *survivor-*

ship work in part by giving expression to some ambiguities associated with the cancer diagnosis. Most patients desperately want some hope for cure and relief from fear. Like the term *complete remission*, which sounds like cure, *survivor* and *survivorhood* suggest that cancer is in the past, behind them. But if we had really meant to signal certainty about cure, we would talk about people who had cancer in the past or who were *cured* of their cancer (there were cured cancer clubs in the early twentieth century). While this ambiguity and fuzziness can be useful and understandable in some situations, there are costs. Optimistic distortions of prognosis among the very ill can lead to unnecessarily aggressive or futile treatment and its attendant physical and financial harms. At the other end, the quadrupling of people labeled as cancer survivors in recent decades can lead to the perception that screening, surveillance, and preventative treatment are effective while the expansion might have very little to do with greater efficacy and a lot to do with an increase in the numbers of people diagnosed. Obscuring the meaning of the cancer experience is also a challenge to the long-established ethical obligation to speak truthfully to patients.

The cancer survivorship movement has valorized the person with cancer. But this valorization is thin if it is based simply on the brute fact of continued life after the cancer diagnosis. Personal agency in "outliving" cancer is often exaggerated and ignores the role of screening, diagnostic expansion, and greatly expanded prevalence and risk states in shaping apparent success. And the valorization of cancer survivorship begs the question of how much and what we value about survival, especially when there are difficult trade-offs between the harms of medical treatment and the often small chances they may extend life's duration. These are questions many patients with progressive cancer confront, especially as the course of cancer and failure of treatment sometimes force them to recalibrate their hopes from escaping death to finding meaning in a life fraught with pain, uncertain decisions, and declining function.

8

The global circulation of
risk interventions

One day in 1988, while I was working as a doctor in a rural Tanzanian hospital, a van pulled up and let out a few South Asian men carrying a film projector. To a group of nurses and medical assistants assembled for morning rounds, they showed a crude English-language movie promoting the benefits of an injectable iron medicine produced by an Indian pharmaceutical company. They left after perfunctorily answering a few questions. I do not recall who invited them, the exact product they were selling, or the reactions of the assembled group.[1] But I do remember the absurdity of the situation.

Then or now there is almost no clinical utility for injectable iron either in Tanzania or the U.S. If an individual is iron deficient and has a functioning gastrointestinal tract, oral iron is safe, cheap, and effective. If patients are acutely and dangerously anemic, then they need blood transfusions. And whether hawking a useless or essential drug, what were American-style pharmaceutical "detail men" doing in remote Tanzania, where there was no apparent purchaser of drugs? Our hospital pharmacy was stocked almost entirely with medicines donated from abroad.

As an inexperienced volunteer physician on a short-term stay, I was only vaguely aware at that time of the cash and barter economy of medications entered into by patients and their families outside the hospital. Nor did I know anything about the value that some East Africans placed on injectable medications.[2] But now knowing these and other realities, the injectable iron medicine show appears as a harbinger of a global pharmaceutical economy that increasingly knits the poorest parts of the globe with middle-income and rich regions.[3]

In these intervening years, I have been researching the intertwined intellectual, social, and material histories of health risks in the U.S. and other industrialized countries. I have become concerned about the possible waste and harm caused by the export of ineffective or only marginally effective but expensive risk-reducing interventions from rich and middle-income regions to poor ones, such as some cardiovascular risk-lowering drugs and cancer-screening tests.[4] Even interventions widely accepted as efficacious and safe in the global north may work differently when adopted in other regions because efficacy and safety are in part locally constituted, not solely the result of standardized practices or products triggering universal physiological responses.

Let me say at the outset that risk interventions, like other health practices, often have complicated origins, can vary widely within regions (for example, different national practices about cancer screening within Western Europe and the U.S.), and the flow of diverse ideas, products, and practices can go in many directions (north-south, south-north, south-south, and within regions and localities). But at the same time, under the umbrella of global health, international health organizations, influential nongovernmental groups, and large national and multinational pharmaceutical companies are often promoting and testing interventions in multiple regions of the world, resulting in a largely center-to-periphery flow.

Many of my concerns about the global circulation of risk-reducing practices have understandably received little attention. The major health problems facing poor countries are caused by socioeconomic problems and inadequate clinical and public health infrastructure—not flawed imported interventions against health risks.[5] It is nevertheless worthwhile to explore some nascent or emerging problems in the global circulation of risk-reducing interventions, as the challenges they pose may become more significant as health care globalizes.

I focus on some recent efforts to prevent cervical cancer in rich, middle-income, and poor parts of the world as presented in published and online business plans, policy deliberations, individual responses to controversies, and research findings. Most of this material concerns trial runs of "see and treat" programs, the new HPV vaccines, and HPV DNA screening tests.[6] In addition, I briefly examine pharmaceutical interventions in type 2 diabetes, a diagnosis that has elements of both a risk state and a symptomatic chronic disease, and some tensions that exist between national and international vaccine policies.

I also raise a more general concern about how health risks that emerge from commodities (e.g., the cigarette) and patterns of consumption (e.g., high caloric intake) are vigorously exported from countries with excess production and marketing capacity, while the clinical, public health, and policy responses that have moderated the impact of these risks are not so easily exported or replicated. As a result, global health inequalities can be exacerbated.

Many risk-reducing drugs, e.g., cholesterol, glucose, or blood pressure lowering—are poised for export or for widespread manufacture and marketing because they have low marginal production costs, are highly palatable, and easily transported. There is also great demand—and potential to create even more demand—for practices and products that promise to prevent disease, especially in societies (or strata within them) in which the research and clinical infrastructure and trained personnel to treat disease are absent or inadequate.

Despite this appeal, the global circulation of risk-reducing interventions can be problematic. For example, the physical structure, potency, and other material properties of some risk-reducing medications are shaped by their origins in rich countries. Their export to poorer parts of the globe can result in a mismatch with the health problems on the ground because medical, social, and economic conditions are different. Risk-reducing practices and products can also divert attention and resources from more pressing social and medical problems as well as nonmedical means of promoting health. Despite the promise of more effective prevention, the diffusion of many risk-reducing practices and products in resource-poor settings can lead to overtreatment and inefficiencies.[7] They can deprivilege the status of practitioners and local medical knowledge.[8]

There is also, of course, an important potential upside to risk intervention—preventing disease, thereby relieving suffering and saving lives. And skepticism towards the expansion of risk-reducing practices and products is in all likelihood not the attitude of many health care providers and laypersons living in poor regions. They may understandably want what people in richer regions have and be rightly

suspicious of double standards. The promise of prevention and expectations of equal treatment are nevertheless even more reason to
critically examine the global circulation of risk ideas and interventions, as the gap between promise and expectation and actual practice
can be significant.

Local origins, global use

Differences between the historical, social, and economic contexts in
which risk interventions originate and the contexts in which they are
later used can lead to unanticipated health consequences. Some recent examples are the new HPV vaccines, whose architecture and cost
constrain their promise to reduce the harms of cervical cancer in poor
parts of the world.[9] Cervical cancer is a very real problem in rich and
poor countries alike. In the U.S. in 2009, National Cancer Institute
officials estimated there were 11,270 new cases of invasive cervical
cancer and 4,070 deaths.[10] There were significant racial and socioeconomic disparities. African American women, for example, had over
twice the chance of developing invasive cervical cancer and over three
times the risk of dying from the disease than white women.[11] These
rates were nevertheless a very small fraction of the total burden of
suffering from cancer in the U.S. The problem is far worse in some
poor countries, where women have been dying from cervical cancer
at seven times the rate of women in rich countries, making it a leading cause of cancer death, and rates are if anything increasing, driven
in many places by the lethal interaction between HIV and HPV infections.[12]

Given this burden of disease, many people have urged that HPV
vaccines be made available in the global south. But the existing vaccines were designed for a very different population. As discussed in
chapter 5, these products—their architecture, manufacturing details,
marketing, and cost—have features of risk-reducing pharmaceuticals
as well as traditional vaccines. They are cost-effective in rich countries
not so much by reducing the harm caused by warts and cervical cancer but by reducing the number of abnormal Pap smears (some three
million women in the U.S. are diagnosed yearly with ASCUS, atypical
squamous cells of uncertain significance). The workup and manage-

ment of these abnormal tests consumes billions of dollars, and the vaccines are likely to dramatically reduce the number of abnormal tests, as many abnormalities are caused by infection from the HPV types included in the vaccines.

The current HPV vaccines licensed in Europe and the U.S., Merck's Gardasil and GlaxoSmithKline's Cervarix, share ingenious and expensive-to-produce viral-like particles (VLPs) that provoke immunological reactions to HPV types 16 and 18.[13] In Europe and North America, these two HPV types are associated with some 70 percent of existing cervical cancer.

The potential contribution of other HPV variants to cervical cancer did not push either of these vaccine makers to initially target them in their vaccines.[14] Reasons for not adding HPV types include their increased cost and concern with possible side effects. Vaccine development is also a stepwise, costly, time-consuming process, so the initial development of vaccines targeting the most pathogenic strains inevitably constrained later developments. But these factors (discussed in more detail below) give an incomplete picture of the market and medical logic of an HPV vaccine developed for economically advanced regions. The existing vaccines were *efficacious enough* in places where cervical cancer is not a leading cause of cancer mortality, the vaccines' efficacy in reducing mortality would be hard to see and measure, other means of prevention exist, and the vaccines could be marketed to individuals as risk-reducing products (see chapter 5).

While HPV vaccines are already reducing the prevalence of precancerous lesions in the U.S., the additional cervical cancer mortality benefit to existing Pap smear screening followed by treatment will take more time to measure.[15] It remains to be seen, for example, whether nontargeted HPV types will prove more pathogenic in vaccinated populations once persistent infection from HPV types included in the vaccine is prevented.[16]

In Western markets, the current HPV vaccines resemble risk-reducing drugs like statins in addition to their identity as cancer-preventing vaccines. HPV vaccines are produced by the latest recombinant DNA technology. As a result, manufacturers may more easily obtain patent protection for them than for traditional vaccines produced via less standardized biological processes.[17] These new vaccines were constructed and marketed to appeal to market segments rather

than having a self-evident life-saving rationale for the whole population (e.g., Merck added wart-causing HPV VLPs to appeal to the male
segment) and reflect no commitment to population goals like herd
immunity. They have been priced high and marketed in direct-to-
consumer advertisements with catchy names, rather than having their
access shaped by public health agencies. For individual consumers,
the vaccines promise to control fears of cancer, stigma, and defile-
ment from a sexually transmitted disease as much as prevention of
their biological target condition, HPV-induced cancers. As I argue in
chapter 5, the vaccines have been marketed to reduce the work and
hassle of living in a constant state of risk from testing positive for HPV
infection.

So we are in a deeply paradoxical situation. HPV vaccines have been
marketed in rich countries where their most predictable economic impact will be to reduce the iatrogenic harm and costs of existing screening programs and their efficacy against cervical cancer mortality may
be small and difficult to perceive. But the vaccines are not generally
available in poor countries where the burden of cervical cancer is so
much higher and the potential to save lives much greater. The current price of the vaccines alone prohibits their widespread use in many
poor countries.

This imbalance is widely recognized, and there are a few access programs designed to get HPV vaccines to poor and middle-income countries. One such early program was funded by Merck, the manufacturer
of Gardasil.[18] In addition to believing it is the right thing to do if there
were no associated costs, providing Gardasil to poor countries can create much needed goodwill for Merck, important for gaining access to
markets for drugs that stand to produce profits. Some middle-income
countries, like India and Brazil, contain growing middle classes that
can already afford to pay for many of Merck's products (as well as those
produced by their burgeoning domestic pharmaceutical companies).
But these countries, let alone some neighboring ones, also contain extremely poor people who have great medical needs but cannot afford
medications. So a balancing act is often required of pharmaceutical
companies: providing some drugs to the poor free or at cost in order
to facilitate the profitable sale of others.[19]

Although HPV 16 and 18 appear throughout the world and account
for the majority of cervical cancer cases, there are global differences

in their contribution and the role played by other types. Mostly we do not know which HPV types are implicated in cervical cancer etiology in poor parts of the world because extensive basic research has not been done there. And accurate data are unlikely because they would require widespread clinical monitoring and tumor registries, infrastructure generally lacking in resource-poor parts of the world. One study found that cervical cancer incident cases are attributed to HPV 16 and 18 in 63.9 percent of sub-Saharan African cases as opposed to 71.5 percent of European/North American cases. HPV 45 appears to be more prevalent in sub-Saharan Africa than anywhere else in the world as well as possibly being causally associated with cervical cancer. Because of these and other differences as well as lack of precise knowledge, some observers had called for including the seven most common HPV types associated with cervical cancer in vaccines, arguing that it was technically possible to create vaccines that could prevent 90 percent rather than 70 percent of HPV-related cancers.[20] Vaccine manufacturers reportedly acknowledged that including additional HPV types in vaccines would not produce interference but "creates more manufacturing difficulties and costs."[21]

Such vaccines are now under development. Could a vaccine have been produced earlier that was a better fit with the cervical cancer problem as it exists in poor countries? Harald zur Hausen, who received the Nobel Prize in Medicine for his role in discovering the HPV-cancer link, had argued a decade ago for more serious consideration to developing a vaccine from more "traditional recombinant proteins," which might be both effective and more affordable than the currently used VLP vaccines.[22]

There have not only been financial, technical, and scientific obstacles to initially developing a more effective vaccine for poorer parts of the world; the inertia and path dependency of earlier choices also plays a role. Technologies develop in particular social, cultural, and economic contexts. Once the technologies are produced, the values and priorities that reflect their local origins are often obscured as they travel far from their place of origin. Technologies may become successful not only for their superior quality or fit but because of the high costs of unseating them.[23] So while a good deal of attention has been given to how we might finance and distribute current HPV vaccines in poor countries via access programs, until recently little attention has been given to the way that the provenance of these vaccines in rich countries has led to an architecture and materiality—e.g., their expensive and high-tech manufacture and limited HPV serotype targets—that make them less than ideal for preventing HPV-related disease in poor countries. These countries need a vaccine that is more than *efficacious enough*.[24]

So far, however, only the two vaccines that target the two main cancer-associated HPV types have been licensed in the U.S. and used in both poor and rich regions of the world. Clinical, economic, social, and cultural factors in Western societies have shaped these vaccines' architecture and scientific and social efficacy as well as their high costs of production and development. While these vaccines are generally understood to be the right tools to prevent cervical cancer, they look less right the further one gets from the societies from which they emerged.

NGOs with international reach have made some initial efforts to disseminate the existing HPV vaccines, whether they are the best tools or not, in poorer parts of the non-Western world. One of the most ambitious efforts to date has come from PATH (Program for Appropriate Technology in Health), a large decades-old Seattle-based NGO active in promoting the production and use of health technologies in poor regions of the globe. While originally most active in contraceptive technology, PATH in recent years has been a leader in vaccines and vaccine-delivery technologies and practices. With Bill and Melinda Gates Foundation funding, in the late 2000s it began an ambitious program to bring HPV vaccines to poor parts of the globe. But its four-country HPV vaccine "demonstration project" very quickly became embroiled in controversy in India, becoming an international news story in the summer of 2013 when an Indian parliamentary committee issued a highly critical report.[25]

This controversy highlights another set of consequences of the global circulation of risk interventions. Mass risk interventions depend on trust. As I described in chapter 3, trust in their safety and efficacy is inextricably connected to the credibility and authority of the groups which have a hand in promoting their use, in this case public health officials, NGOs, pharmaceutical companies, and governmental regulators. In the U.S., a complex process fought out in the pages of

medical journals and the media, within regulatory bodies and professional organizations, resulted in governmental permission to market
HPV vaccines, endorsement by expert advisory boards, and general
but by no means universal acceptance by practitioners and the lay
public. But these tenuous judgments and compromises do not necessarily travel very well and trust in public health authorities, regulatory bodies, NGOs, and pharmaceutical companies can easily unravel
in new settings.

The HPV vaccine controversy in India followed partly from the
immense health care disparities that exist there. Large segments of
India's population are affluent and have access to the latest in medical
technologies and practices, often in five-star hospitals that also cater
to affluent foreigners from nearby poor countries and globally (as
they can often provide much-sought-out high-tech care less expen-
sively than in Western countries). This reality coexists with resource-
starved government- and charity-provided care. These disparities are
not only very visible but are lived out by medical practitioners who
often simultaneously work within these different medical worlds.

The HPV vaccines in India have traveled along these fractured fault
lines, gaining regulatory approval in India for use (after medical licen-
sure in the U.S. and other Western countries) by paying or insured
patients within the first-class system of care while PATH had already
begun to "test" its vaccine giveaway program in two very poor regions
(Vadodara in Gujarat, and Khammam in Andhra Pradesh), an arrange-
ment brokered between PATH and the Indian Council for Medical Research (ICMR).[26]

Controversy over this "demonstration project" was only indirectly
connected to the vaccines' effectiveness, safety, or cost. It was mostly
over the "fishy" (the term used by the Indian parliamentary committee
reviewing developments) entanglements of Western NGOs, the pharmaceutical industry, and the Indian governmental bodies charged
with regulating drug and vaccine use. The fishiness detected by the
Indian parliamentarians underscores the way some routine business
and medical and public health practices developed originally in some
Western countries can breed suspicion and lack of trust as these practices migrate.[27] Their everyday contradictions are perhaps made more
visible in a different context, especially those between high-minded

rhetoric and goals of disease prevention and immunization and the profit to be gained by securing national, regional, and global markets for mass health risk interventions.

PATH officials seemed genuinely bewildered by the controversy that enveloped this attempt to get an effective prevention product to people who needed it. Many reports focused on claims that a small number of child suicides were caused by the vaccine. As these claims were unsubstantiated and causality difficult to prove, it was relatively easy for PATH officials and program supporters to dismiss them as scientifically ignorant, and to suggest nefarious motivations for focusing on them.[28]

Yet even a cursory examination of the strident Indian parliamentary report that investigated the HPV vaccine rollout in these two poor regions suggests that the controversy had little to do with the vaccine's putative role in causing suicide or other direct side effects of vaccination. Instead, the committee focused on ethical issues related to this "experimental" program and what they perceived was a lion (multinational pharmaceutical companies poised to profit from these vaccines once established as commodities and public health vehicles) in sheep's clothing (as sponsor of vaccine giveaway programs).

The central and unifying accusation in the parliamentary report was the heavy-handed and misleading ways a supposed experiment designed to test the vaccine's safety and efficacy in India (the committee's, not PATH's, characterization of these practices) was from top to bottom a *marketing effort* to increase the sales of Gardasil and Cervarix and eventually lead to their being mandated and paid for by government authorities. The parliamentarians were upset by the underhanded and stealthy goal of creating a large market in India for the financial gain of pharmaceutical companies.

The parliamentary committee noted that the trial's purpose was not to test the vaccine's safety and efficacy but to (in PATH's own words) "generate and disseminate evidence for informed public sector introduction of HPV vaccines."[29] The parliamentarians dismissed or ignored PATH's assertion that the vaccine's efficacy and safety had already been established in globalized clinical trials and by regulatory review in the U.S. and elsewhere. PATH's self-description of its practices as an "observational study" was characterized as evasive, even though from PATH's perspective this formulation was an accurate, if somewhat euphemistic way of describing their social marketing efforts (as well as postmarketing surveillance).

The parliamentary committee criticized the inadequate informed consent within a project that exposed a vulnerable population of 23,000 ten- to fourteen-year-old girls to a product that some believed represented a potential health hazard. Over 2,000 consent forms were signed by proxies such as school officials and the many of the remaining forms were initialed by a parent's fingerprints.

However, since from PATH's perspective, the only "experiment" was to figure out the best way to get these vaccines into the bodies of poor rural Indians, allegations of inadequate informed consent seemed beside the point. As the vaccine program was not really an experiment, PATH officials saw no need to closely hew to standard human subject protections. From their perspective, these vaccines' safety and efficacy had already been established in globalized clinical trials. And there was also nothing unseemly in their efforts to rapidly expand the markets for these vaccines. When you are marketing safe and effective vaccines, why not use any and all known techniques from consumer marketing to build a large and stable demand for them?

However, from the more skeptical vantage point of the Indian parliamentary committee, PATH's goal was to manipulate India's public health authorities into adopting practices profitable to the pharmaceutical industry but not necessarily the public's health. According to the parliamentary report, the four countries targeted by PATH (India, Uganda, Peru, and Vietnam) were chosen to reach each of the major ethnic groups that "reside in developing countries. Such data would be invaluable to promote the two branded, patented, single source HPV vaccine all over the world." It also did not escape the committee's attention that each of these countries has "state-funded national vaccine immunization programs." The committee objected to Merck's and SKB's monopoly of the HPV market, generating windfall profits, and viewed the PATH program as part of their "well planned scheme to commercially exploit a situation." Overall, "the committee finds the entire matter very intriguing and fishy."[30]

Additional parliamentary criticism was directed at the lax regulation of PATH by Indian medical authorities who were depicted as kowtowing to American NGOs and corporate interests. The committee believed that the ICMR "lent its platform to PATH in an improper and unlawful manner."[31] The committee criticized ICMR for its inadequate plans for reporting and responding to adverse events, noting that ICMR worried more about the bad publicity that might emanate from reports of side effects rather than the side effects themselves. Moreover, the involvement of ICMR, rather than more appropriate Indian regulatory bodies (National Technological Advisory Group on Immunization), was in itself evidence of shady behavior.[32]

According to the parliamentary committee, the oversight of PATH practices was riddled with conflicts of interest. For example, India's Ministry of Health and Family Welfare did the initial inquiry into the controversy. The ministry selected a group of "highly learned members" to conduct this inquiry. Members were supposed to be above reproach, but the parliamentary committee rebuffed this claim by randomly selecting one of the members and checking to see if there were any potential conflicts of interest. The committee quickly discovered that this individual had received money from Merck to research the proper dosage of Gardasil.

The parliamentary committee had perceived a scandal that was constituted by conflict of interest and very aggressive marketing practices. One can understand the concern that might emanate from realizing that drug companies, rather than some independent and objective third party, create and analyze the very data used to regulate their products, as is the case in the U.S. and elsewhere.

Throughout this controversy, committee members saw PATH initiatives through the lens of Merck's or SKB's marketing of other drugs in India, by their "whatever it takes" full-court press to increase pharmaceutical revenues and market share by manipulating Indian regulatory bodies and other heavy-handed actions. There is a great deal of existing mistrust of domestic and international pharmaceutical companies and their collusion with corrupt and/or incompetent domestic regulatory agencies. Ultimately the success of any mass clinical or public health program depends on trust among the different stakeholders. This is why practices that can undermine trust are consequential, even if it is the perception of motivations and goals, more than the efficacy and safety of products, that dominates the controversy.

One of the most visible examples of aggressive marketing of Western pharmaceutics in India, one that illustrates additional challenges posed by the global circulation of risk interventions, are medications

against type 2 diabetes. The pharmaceutical treatment of type 2 diabetes is not so much aimed at treating symptoms of an active chronic
disease (there may or may not be excessive urination and dehydration;
more often the condition is diagnosed among the asymptomatic by
laboratory testing or becomes asymptomatic after initial treatment)
but reducing the risk of infections and different types of end organ
damage, especially to the cardiovascular system, kidneys, and eyes.
As an asymptomatic risk state with a flexible definition, the market
for diabetes medications in rich and poor countries is large and ex-
pandable.

Because of its large population, increasing obesity, and other
trends, India can claim the dubious honor of having the world's largest
population of diabetics. Merck has aggressively marketed Januvia, one
of its newer diabetes drugs, in India over the past few years. Januvia
was one of the first drugs protected by Western patents that successfully found a toehold in the Indian market.[33] The rationale for treating
chronic disease is self-evident, but it is less well appreciated that pharmaceutical companies' promotion of drugs like Januvia also can also
transform, and contribute to the shift to, chronic disease, by increasing the numbers of people diagnosed and widening the spectrum of
disease. Pharmaceutical companies often promote a highly medicalized, risk-inflected, transmuted chronic disease as well as products to
treat them—i.e., the target condition, asymptomatic type 2 diabetes,
and the interventions against it are sold together.[34]

In Western markets, Januvia is a second- or third-line drug for
type 2 diabetics. It works by a new mechanism, inhibiting DPP-4,
an enzyme that degrades insulin. This novel mechanism makes the
drug appealing to clinicians because Januvia can be used on top of
older drugs that work by different mechanisms. Merck used innovative "rapid fire" marketing to quickly get Januvia a significant share of
the very large and expanding worldwide diabetes market.[35] In India,
Merck decided to price the drug at one-fifth its price in the U.S. and
Europe, a necessary step to gain market share in India but one that invited criticism of price gouging in Western markets. Januvia's aggressive marketing meant that it was likely to be tried sooner rather than
later in a patient's personal history of diabetes.[36]

The rapid deployment of a new, expensive risk-reducing medication is problematic in high-income countries, let alone middle-income

ones. Diabetes is a complex risk state. The efficacy of diabetes drugs for an individual is usually determined by easily measured endpoints such as serum glucose and HgA1c levels. These are short and slightly longer term measures of hyperglycemia (high "sugar" levels in the blood), but the more clinically relevant endpoint is whether a diabetes drug prevents infections and end organ damage—stroke, heart disease, kidney disease, etc. This long-term efficacy must additionally be measured against the short- and long-term effects of the drug itself. It takes a long time, careful study, and large numbers of people to evaluate long-term efficacy and safety. Unfortunately, many drugs for adult-onset diabetes that have appeared to significantly impact short- and intermediate-term endpoints, when subjected to long-term clinical trials, have turned out to be less efficacious than imagined, not efficacious, or even dangerous.[37]

For these reasons, Januvia's long-term scientific efficacy and safety will take time to evaluate.[38] The drug's rapid diffusion in India, following on the heels of extensive and innovative marketing, is especially problematic because India has relatively less capacity than the U.S. and Western European countries for surveillance and regulation (although as a boisterous democracy with a very active press, there is no shortage of potential lay and political opposition to medical practices suspected of having flaws—as in HPV vaccine controversy discussed above). In India, there is little infrastructure to pick up and report adverse drug reactions. In this setting, there arguably should be even more therapeutic caution than in richer countries towards new drugs, especially those which promise primary or secondary prevention of chronic disease, because the benefits are so easily hyped and so difficult to measure.[39]

A final example of the challenges posed by the global circulation of risk-reducing interventions is a product that problematically *did not* travel from rich to poor countries. RotaShield, a vaccine against rotavirus infection, a leading cause of diarrhea globally, was tested in clinical trials starting in the late 1980s, and was successfully shepherded through regulatory bureaucracy and marketed in the U.S. in the late 1990s. However, a few cases of intussusception, a dangerous condition in which one part of the intestine slides into the next, were reported following vaccination and linked to the vaccine.

Because of its demonstrated efficacy and yet a small if uncertain risk of intussusception, U.S. regulators faced a difficult decision about whether to withdraw the vaccine. In the U.S., rotavirus infection rarely led to infant deaths (in part because of the availability of medical care), so even a small probability of a serious medical risk might negate the benefits of the vaccine. Moreover, there was an understandable concern among policy makers that continued use of this vaccine would damage public trust in the safety of the entire vaccine enterprise, a worry made more immediate by the concurrent and very public controversies over autism and MMR vaccines.

Regulators decided to pull the vaccine from the market, although some voiced concern at the time about the impact of that decision on the fate of the vaccine in the global south, where the benefits of the vaccine in preventing infant mortality far outweighed the small risks of intussusception. Although the regulatory problem was explicitly about the U.S. only, regulators knew that poorer countries, despite the different risk-benefit reality, would likely follow suit and never deploy the vaccine once it was withdrawn from U.S. markets.[40] But like the marketing and development of the technology itself, regulatory practice gives understandable priority to the local. The consequences, however, can and have been global.

When risks and efforts to tame them circulate unequally

In an interconnected world, the way affluent societies experience and tame health risks—in terms of timing, adaptation, and response—can profoundly impact poorer societies or poorer people within richer societies. This is especially true of risks that emanate from changing economic and material conditions.

In some respects, the current global exchange of health risks and risk interventions recapitulates the well-known narrative that connects technological progress and global commerce to the spread of infectious diseases in both the recent and distant past. Cholera became pandemic in the nineteenth century and AIDS in the twentieth century partly because of improved global trade and transportation. While pandemic, these diseases have impacted rich and poor societies very differently. Cholera epidemics recur periodically in the global south, including Haiti and Zimbabwe in recent years, while they have been effectively banished in the global north since the late nineteenth century. Not only has there been greater availability of effective AIDS treatment in the global north, but the greater affluence and gender equality has contributed to different patterns of HIV transmission and prevalence. Moreover, economic inequality between north and south can directly contribute to disease transmission. It is not just the poverty of Haiti, but its poverty relative to its proximal northern neighbor; this enabled a thriving sex tourism industry, which amplified the HIV epidemic early on.[41] And the health consequences of severe chronic infections like AIDS and tuberculosis further exacerbates—via decreased productivity and resources devoted to the care of the ill and dying—the economic gap between rich and poor societies, creating conditions for more economic and health inequality.

In the more distant past, highly developed agricultural societies' different and earlier biological experience with specific infectious diseases had profound impacts on lesser developed ones. The most dramatic historical example followed from the earlier adoption of agriculture in the Middle East and Europe, the resulting increase in population density, and the concomitant domestication of large animals. These developments, which led to close animal-human contact and transfer of germs, were important proximal causes of the emergence of many animal-originating epidemic diseases. These societies' long history with diseases we now recognize as smallpox, measles, and others has led over time to the situation in which the population damage these diseases caused, while severe, did not threaten them with extinction. Smallpox epidemics led to many deaths but also to life-long immunity for those who survived—and probably exerted a selective force favoring the reproductive success of individuals with some immune or other resistance. In addition, inoculation was practiced in Asia since the Middle Ages and was incompletely adopted by European societies, mitigating the population impact of the disease. Measles and some other infectious diseases were transformed over time into childhood diseases, from which many children survived with lifelong immunity. As a result of this history, the process of European colonization of the New World involved the unequal—in terms of population impact certainly—exchange of infectious disease and populations with different levels of immunity, perhaps the most devastating impact of colonization even if the least premeditated and immoral.[42]

Today there may be a new global exchange of disease and risk, one mediated more by commodities and patterns of consumption than by infectious agents. A more affluent society's earlier experience with and ability to tame consumption-related health risks creates hazards for poorer societies in ways similar to the Columbian exchange of germs and unequally immune populations, even if the mechanisms are completely different and the collision of populations is less direct.

Many noninfectious health risks that emanate from social and material conditions, such as cigarette use, high-fat diet, and increasing sedentariness, were initially more prevalent among the more affluent within rich societies. But better-off people were often able to develop social, intellectual, and material responses that mediated the impact of these risks. Risks then become relatively more prevalent among the less affluent due to successful evasion among people with resources and greater uptake or exposure to risk among poorer people due to class dynamics and other factors.[43] Such shifts occurred with coronary heart disease and some tobacco-related illnesses in the U.S. throughout the twentieth century. Starting in the 1960s, there was a general decline in cardiovascular disease in developed countries, leaving in its wake a more stratified picture in which people of lesser means bore more of the disease burden.

This pattern also exists between rich and poor regions of the world. While commodities-as-risks easily circulate, the infrastructure, knowledge, and resources that enabled the more affluent to effectively respond to or evade them, e.g., laws that limit tobacco advertising or require food labeling, are often not exported as easily. The earlier exposure to and knowledge of health risks in rich societies can create the situation in which risks from consumption are tamed, or relatively better tamed, and then are exported and diffused to groups who will experience greater harm because they lack the social and economic capital to protect themselves in the ways that richer societies have done. In some cases, such as alcohol use and diabetes among some indigenous Americans, there may also be greater genetic and social predispositions that exacerbate the impact of these risks. In many such modern-day exchanges, the power and indifference of commercial interests sustain and exacerbate the negative health consequences of many exchanges of risks and risk interventions.

Perhaps the best example here is the cigarette, but alcohol, nutrition-challenged foods, and aspects of the built environment that sustain sedentary lifestyle raise similar issues.[44] Carefully documented by Allan Brandt in *The Cigarette Century*, tobacco companies in the U.S. throughout the twentieth century tinkered with tobacco delivery mechanisms and nicotine content while mass marketing the cigarette as youthful, a symbol of nonconformity, and modern. As a result, the cigarette diffused widely through American society, starting with more affluent men but eventually to all classes and women. As the health consequences of tobacco were recognized, this market expansion eventually met with decades of public health and lay opposition that has made serious inroads into tobacco addiction in the U.S. and other affluent countries, although leaving in its wake a much more socially stratified distribution of tobacco use.

With markets limited in Western countries, and with decades of marketing and production experience, tobacco companies have sought global markets. As a result, cigarette consumption is rapidly rising in China, India, and elsewhere, creating conditions for lung cancer, cardiovascular disease, and respiratory failure throughout the world. Brandt documented how both domestic and international attempts to limit this expansion have been blocked by tobacco companies and the U.S. government, which have added to their traditional arguments against tobacco regulation the more effective one for our age—that setting limits on tobacco marketing is an infringement of global trade and constitutes a form of protectionism.[45]

Less is more? "Appropriate" technologies and practices and their global circulation

Health officials and health care workers, NGOs, and academic researchers in the global south have long recognized that the best and most practical ways to prevent disease will not necessarily be the ones that work in the global north. There has also been an intense debate in recent decades about which medications are effective and give good value for money and should therefore be seen as essential to health everywhere, i.e., the movement to specify and find ways of providing *essential medicines* globally.[46] Foundations like the Gates Foundation are committed to finding new interventions that are appropriate to the resources, climate, and culture of the "developing" world.[47]

An interesting case of successful practices and technologies that were first developed and promoted in poor regions are the different efforts at early detection and treatment of cervical cancer. The direction of innovation has not been simply to produce cheaper, more practical, and bare-boned versions of practices and technology used in rich countries, but hybrid "high-tech/low-tech" systems that have the potential to influence practice in the global north.

A considerable amount of effort has gone into devising "appropriate" alternatives to the routine pelvic examination and Pap smear, the principal means of cervical cancer prevention in rich countries (although there are significant differences among rich countries in how these practices are used). The cost and the transportation, medical, and information infrastructure requirements of Pap smear screening have generally precluded its use in poor parts of the world.[48] Routine Pap testing as practiced in, say, Philadelphia depends on access to regular primary care and reliable diagnostic laboratories staffed by trained cytological technicians who are backed up by pathologists, gynecological surgeons prepared to excise abnormal lesions, and communication and information systems connecting patients, doctors, and laboratories.[49]

Once or twice in a lifetime "see and treat" strategies for women in their thirties have been promoted as an efficient and safe alternative way to prevent cervical cancer in poor parts of the world. "See and treat" typically involves health care worker visualization of the cervix, aided by simple staining with acetic acid or Lugol's iodine. If abnormalities suggestive of cervical cancer are seen, then the lesions are frozen (cryotherapy) at the same visit. "See and treat" has shown promise, but its use has been controversial both because its efficacy is contested and some people have objected to providing something less than the standard of care in the U.S.[50]

Over the past few years, researchers have been testing and deploying HPV DNA tests, which detect HPV infection in cervical and vaginal specimens, within the "see and treat" paradigm. In rich countries, there has been only limited use of HPV DNA tests as a stand-alone screening tool. These tests have been mostly used along with more traditional Pap testing, serving as a supplement rather than a replacement for them. In addition to improving the diagnostic accuracy of the Pap smear, HPV DNA tests address a widespread limitation associated with them in rich countries. Technicians sample Pap smears and scan them for cellular abnormalities. If technicians suspect they have found an abnormality, they then seek confirmation from a pathologist. It is not surprising that this nonspecific, probabilistic, needle-in-a-haystack means of detection can miss some cancers and high-risk lesions while at the same time producing many false positives. As a consequence, Pap tests have become the subject of many "failure to diagnose" malpractice lawsuits. This legal climate is one important reason why HPV DNA tests, whose results are machine read, have found a niche in rich countries alongside Pap testing. They remove a lot of the human operator element, whose failure forms the crux of malpractice suits. This efficacy, reducing physician and laboratory malpractice liability, has, of course, little to no meaning in poor parts of the world.

Given this aspect of efficacy within rich countries and the high cost of the test, the HPV DNA test does not seem a likely candidate for use in resource-poor areas.[51] But it has been used and evaluated as part of once- or twice-in-a-lifetime "see and treat" programs among older women. Unlike Pap smear interpretation, HPV DNA tests can be evaluated without cytotechnicians and pathologists, although it requires laboratory analysis. Since this laboratory analysis takes time to process (although portable, rapid tests are now being deployed), the treat step of "see and treat" for women who test positive is neither immediate nor done under direct visualization. Instead, health care workers usually carry out "blind" cryotherapy (resulting in some overtreatment) or freeze lesions localized by acetic acid or iodine in women who test positive for HPV.

This hybrid high-tech/low-tech strategy made international news when the surprising results of a study of its effectiveness in India were reported in the *New England Journal of Medicine* in 2009.[52] This study showed that once-in-a-lifetime HPV screening, followed by cervical visualization and treatment, was effective at reducing cervical cancer mortality while the simpler and less expensive acetic acid stains were not.[53] The lack of efficacy of the simpler technique provoked some consternation and puzzlement.[54] This result was not only at odds with other studies that suggested that "see and treat" approaches using acetic acid were effective, but it represented a flip-flop of results reported earlier by the same authors. There was a "man bites dog" aspect to a high-tech test, developed in the West, which has limited utility there in part because of the efficacy of lower cost and more accurate solutions, being more effective and cheaper (since it is used as part of a one-time, not annual or biennial process) when used in poor parts of the world.[55]

In this study, screening was offered to women once and at older ages, taking advantage of what is known about the natural history of cervical cancer. Cervical cancer is slow growing and often can be cured in relatively late stages. Most HPV infections are transient and never result in cancer, although they may take months or years to clear. In those women who will ultimately suffer invasive cervical cancer, HPV infection is usually persistent. At later ages, women have had time to either develop and recover from transient HPV infection or have chronic infection and/or cervical cancer, resulting in greater specificity for HPV DNA tests. Yet severe and difficult-to-treat cervical cancer may still take many years to develop. So the HPV DNA technology, even if deployed among women many years after their initial HPV exposure, may be a test with good enough sensitivity and specificity to find women early enough in their individual history of cervical cancer who would benefit from immediate treatment.[56] In some countries such as India, there are also claims that initial sexual activity occurs at later ages, extending the average age at which cervical cancer will develop, giving yet another reason why once-in-a-lifetime HPV DNA screening of older women might work well. And this technology works while retaining its portability and mechanical objectivity.

The promotion of "see and treat," with or without these HPV DNA tests, has ignited a good deal of controversy. Suba and colleagues have led the skeptical charge against researchers and members of the ACCP (Alliance for Cervical Cancer Prevention) who have promoted simpler "see and treat" programs globally, pointing out the unfairness of providing less to poorer people. They have argued that "see and treat" is not only less efficacious than Pap testing but also leads to overtreatment. Confronted with arguments that Pap screening is unaffordable and the required infrastructure unattainable in most poor places, Suba and colleagues counter that costs are exaggerated and that cytology infrastructure has been successfully built in some middle-income countries (recall that antiretroviral treatment against AIDS was once thought impossible in resource-poor settings). Suba and colleagues have also criticized the Gates Foundation's fascination with developing new techniques and practices for poor parts of the world, when effective practices already exist in richer countries.[57] They view HPV DNA screening as an expensive distraction. "Within the political structures of many developing countries there is genuine lack of support for cervical-cancer prevention efforts," they argue, "which may be further eroded by the questionable conclusion that only an unaffordable screening option [i.e., DNA tests] is better than none at all." Others have criticized the NEJM study that reported that only HPV screening was effective, citing conflict of interest, bias in the HPV screening arm, use of undertrained cytotechnicians, Tuskegee-like ethical misconduct in having a "no screen" control group, and misuse of intention to treat analysis.[58]

A manufacturer of HPV DNA tests (including new rapid ones), Qiagen, has not only promoted its technology in poor parts of the world but has sponsored large Gardasil giveaway programs. It is possible that Qiagen believes that the success of a continuum of HPV-based strategies in poor parts of the world will eventually lead to greater use of HPV DNA screening in richer countries.[59] The momentum in cervical cancer screening in richer countries is to do screening at older ages and at less frequent intervals—approaching some of the conditions of "see and treat" programs in poor countries.[60] One can imagine calls in U.S. and Western Europe to institute higher-specificity late-life HPV tests to "mop up" cases of persistent HPV infection that slipped through the cracks of HPV vaccination and cytological screening.

Moreover, in some poor regions, the self-collection of HPV DNA is being promoted, sidestepping infrastructure limitations and cultural norms that limit the feasibility of vaginal examinations performed by health care workers in health care settings. In rich countries, this kind of practice is in line with the many direct-to-consumer medical tests such as home pregnancy testing. So if the efficacy of self-collection is established in resource-poor regions, one can imagine it influencing practice in richer ones.[61]

The potential for practices developed for poor parts of the world,

especially those that mix high- and low-tech elements, to shape practices in richer parts of the world underscores the complex, intertwined
global system in which risk interventions are tested and promoted. At
the same time, it remains unclear whether these globally circulating
individual-based cancer screening practices will ultimately be effective or end up diverting resources from primary health care, almost
nonexistent cancer treatment programs, and/or interventions aimed
at the social determinants of health.

Conclusion

James Ferguson has described the often thin, exploitative, non-
accountable transnational system of development that subsumes
the globalized biomedical system.[62] The transnational circulation of
highly portable risk-reducing interventions with no or marginal efficacy, or whose efficacy and safety were established under conditions
very different from those where they will later be used, may be one
expanding front of this system.

Many drugs and practices used to prevent and intervene in the
natural history of chronic diseases also change them. They may catalyze the expansion of risk-inflected diagnoses, transforming asymptomatic or minimally symptomatic states, like many cases of type 2
diabetes, into highly intervened-in illnesses. At the same time, many
countries do not have the regulatory, infrastructure, manpower, and
cultural resources with which to survey the population for adverse
effects or evaluate efficacy of such transforming practices and products. These and many other problems associated with the global circulation of health risk interventions arise from global economic and
power imbalances.

In addition to the need for skepticism and caution about deploying new risk-lowering interventions, one modest policy response to
these challenges is to create more knowledge about the efficacy and
safety of risk interventions in the places where they will be used. This
will require investment in health infrastructure and institutions, and
fostering stable clinical conditions in peripheral areas. Feierman has
made a convincing case for more useable locale-specific knowledge
about medical treatments that correspond to the disease experience

and the diagnostic and therapeutic technologies available in resource-poor parts of the world. Supporting such local knowledge production also means privileging local priorities.[63]

There is no reason to assume that the efficacy and safety of a risk intervention or the health impact of particular risks will be identical or similar in different regions. Furthermore, health risks tamed in the global north may have greater negative impact when exported because poorer societies have had neither the time nor resources to adequately control them. At the same time, some effective practices and products that arise in resource-poor settings may have considerable heuristic and practical value for medical and public health practices in more developed societies.

In some cases, e.g., the use of existing HPV vaccines in poor regions or the mass marketing of new, expensive diabetes medications in middle-income countries, the movement of risk interventions to places where they were not originally used has not led to truly new problems so much as made their already existing cost, efficacy, and/or safety problems that much more visible. Similarly, the ensuing controversies often reveal the preexisting deep skepticism felt by many people about the institutions that regulate medical practices and products and the companies that market them. Whether mediated directly or by uncovering problems already there, the encounter between risk interventions believed to be universally applicable and local epidemiological, economic, and political conditions has led to major challenges that have been under recognized and incompletely addressed.

III

9

Situating health risks: An opportunity for disease prevention policy

The health care issues that capture significant public and professional attention are not necessarily the most important. As potential points of policy intervention, some intellectual assumptions, clinical practices, and structural relationships are so tightly woven into social, economic, and scientific life that they are in some sense invisible.

Take, for example, one of the most contentious American health policy controversies at the beginning of the twenty-first century— Medicare coverage for prescription medications. Participants in this controversy focused almost exclusively on financial and administrative issues such as cost, the scope of benefits, and the role of private insurers. Seemingly—and strangely—absent from political and policy debates was any mention of which drugs seniors take and why. Neither George W. Bush nor Al Gore, both of whom focused on Medicare prescription coverage in a series of presidential debates in 2000, asked why the elderly were taking so many medicines. But consider that twenty of the forty-six drugs most widely used by the elderly in 2000 in my home state of Pennsylvania were drugs prescribed to treat asymptomatic "risk factors" such as osteoporosis, high cholesterol, and hypertension.[1]

The definition, scope, and significance of many of these health risks, such as the treatment of high serum cholesterol levels in the elderly, were widely contested at the time.[2] In addition, the demand for risk-reducing medications was heavily influenced by direct marketing to consumers, the sometimes exaggerated claims of self-interested parties, and problematic assumptions used in the extrapolation of aggregate data to individual decisions. I believe that the developments leading to this state of affairs represented missed opportunities for policy analysis and intervention. Understanding them as policy issues has the potential to significantly impact both population health and our economic well-being.

The limitations of current disease-prevention policy

The elderly's high use of risk-reducing drugs is but one aspect of a disease-prevention landscape that in recent decades has been transformed by social, demographic, economic, intellectual, and technological forces. Yet our traditional mode of making health policy—from FDA regulation of new drugs to expert consensus review of existing clinical practices—is not designed for the challenge posed by the radically changed character, magnitude, and mix of current and future risks and prevention practices. Policy makers have generally responded to the increasing number of newly defined and controversial health risks, screening tests, and risk-reducing drugs long after most have found a secure niche in medical and/or popular ideas and practices. They have not understood developments that occur "upstream" from the time when these prevention ideas and practices take root as potential points of policy intervention. Nor have they adequately grappled with the questions and challenges raised by the nonarbitrary ways that health risks emerge and are responded to. Notably, why have we embraced these risks, drugs, and practices rather than others? Should insurers, purchasers, and regulators intervene to regulate health risk research and scientific and marketplace developments that contribute to the success or failure of new health risk and prevention practices?

Disease prevention policies have generally been based on the critical evaluation of medical evidence about the efficacy and safety of particular screening tests, preventive medications, and calls for behavioral change. Although there has been a great deal of careful evidence-based appraisal of specific preventive policies, and although the ongoing policy response by government and professional groups is in many ways more extensive than the regulation of existing diagnostic and therapeutic practices and technologies, disease-prevention policies have generally been reactive and after-the-fact.

The changed disease prevention landscape is a present concern. Insights derived from the sequencing of the human genome, for example, are already leading to many newly defined genetic "risks" as statistical correlations are made between bits of genomic variation and disease (e.g., breast cancer genes and Alzheimer genes). Such knowledge will inevitably result in many new screening tests, disease classifications, and points of intervention. The pace, shape, and use of these insights and developments are substantially influenced by organizations that finance research, seek patents, and market or franchise genetic tests and preventive measures. It seems myopic to bring the considerable analytic powers of evidence-based medicine to each newly established genetic risk and test without also examining the upstream processes that systematically create these particular risks and risk interventions.

I was reminded of the market significance of new health risks when several pharmaceutical company representatives were waiting to ask me a series of "prediction" questions after I gave a talk on the history of symptoms. I learned that they had attended my talk because they were trying to understand what common symptoms and risks might be the next target for medical interventions—the next Viagra or Premarin. New symptom complexes and health risks are an extremely important frontier for pharmaceutical companies because drugs directed at them have potential markets in the tens of millions and the duration of treatment is often life-long.

We need to find upstream points of policy intervention not just because narrow interests play powerful roles in shaping and responding to health risks or because disease prevention policy is in danger of resembling a complex group process about the best way to close the barn door after the horse has left. We also presumably want our limited research and health care resources to be deployed in ways that target significant health problems and serve the interests of a diverse society. So we need to understand the processes through which we come to recognize and agree about the importance of some health risks and not others.

Take, for example, the political decisions that determine the regulatory options for environmental health risks, such as workplace exposures and industrial pollutants. These options are self-evidently a function of prior funding for surveillance activity by agencies such as the Environmental Protection Agency. We can regulate only those dangerous substances and practices that have been previously recognized, investigated, and named. If there is little financial or logistical support for surveillance practices that identify dangerous exposures and pollutants, then there will be nothing to regulate. Given these links, the very terms of a political and social debate about environmental activism and regulation are often determined by decisions that in themselves are not directly the subject of self-conscious health policy concern.

Debates about the federal regulation of putative environmental carcinogens, for example, depends on earlier surveillance that might identify the cancer-causing agents. Consider that local public health officials are often reluctant to investigate reports of unusual clustering of cancer cases in specific geographic areas because such investigations rarely produce solid evidence of specific causal connections.[3] The aggregate effect of many local decisions not to investigate cancer clusters may be that a smaller number of chemicals will be subject to future regulation. For example, it took a great deal of community pressure and political action to push state health officials to investigate a cancer cluster in New Jersey. This study resulted in the discovery of a new putative environmental carcinogen.[4] Despite the importance of the political and social processes by which knowledge of environmental health risks exists or not, they are not generally deemed relevant to health policy.[5]

Our current health policies have not adequately come to terms with the complex interactions among social factors and biomedical insights that shape our recognition and understanding of health risks and disease prevention practices. In the sections below, I argue why these upstream developments matter and then offer a preliminary sketch of some new areas for disease prevention policy and policy analysis. This type of thought experiment necessarily involves stretching the typical meaning and context of the term *health policy*, which is generally limited to existing means of resource allocation, legislation, regulation, and large-scale decision making.

The natural history of a health risk

It is not at all self-evident why certain health risks attract significant societal and medical attention and become objects of specific prevention practices. It was neither inevitable nor solely determined by biomedical developments, for example, that individuals and groups would search for cancer blood tests in the 1940s,[6] launch large epidemiological studies of "risk factors" for coronary heart disease in the 1950s (chapter 4), abort efforts to screen smokers for cancer in the 1960s,[7] conceptualize posttraumatic stress disorder in the 1970s,[8] launch national cholesterol guidelines in the 1980s,[9] or develop Lyme disease vaccines in the 1990s (chapter 6). We might find more successful policy leverage if we understood the generation-specific and contingent influences on the appearance and identity of risks, diagnoses, and prevention practices.

There are often three stages prior to the widespread diffusion of specific drugs, screening tests, or calls for behavioral change that present opportunities for policy intervention: the *discovery* of the health risk, *making this risk visible* to others, and *creating demand* for specific interventions. While there are no clear boundaries between these stages and many risks and prevention practices have not gone through them in a stepwise manner, this framework can help identify the common elements in the trajectories of disparate health risks as they do or do not elicit specific disease prevention responses.

In the *discovery* stage, individuals and groups first recognize and give a name to new associations among clinical, behavioral, environmental, and laboratory factors and ill health. How does the political and social context in which individuals and groups live affect which risks they identify and label? How have technological changes and the structure of health systems and markets shaped the discovery and naming of health risks?

Elizabeth Armstrong's study of fetal alcohol syndrome (FAS) illustrates some important features of the discovery stage of a health risk.[10] In the early 1970s, activist researchers rediscovered and relabeled older concerns about women, pregnancy, fetuses, and alcohol to construct FAS. Armstrong did not argue that alcohol is safe for the developing fetus, but that the appearance of this new diagnosis was heavily shaped by social influences much more than by research results. Armstrong depicted these activist researchers as "moral entrepreneurs," emphasizing the way they tended to subordinate their own and others' scientific data towards an end about which they had a passionate commitment. These moral entrepreneurs took advantage of, and were influenced by, increased medical interest and progress in classifying birth defects. Armstrong's major concern (and that of much of the historical and sociological literature on health risk discovery) is the way promoters of many twentieth-century health risks (such as fetal alcohol syndrome) reconfigured moral questions—what behaviors are right and wrong, who is and is not responsible for disease—as *seemingly* empirical value-free questions about health risks.

A characteristic feature of this discovery stage has been the way new clinical and pathological insights, frequently driven by new diagnostic technologies, or older ones applied in new circumstances, result in the appearance and naming of novel health risks. The seemingly specific and legitimate associations are often driven by technologies whose reach and limitations are not yet clear (such as ultrasound abnormalities in the early FAS papers) and can thus potentially gain, as I have argued, a good deal of scientific and public traction without (at least in retrospect) adequate scientific review.[11] It often takes a considerable amount of time and tinkering before there are enough data and experiences to evaluate the justification for and strength of initial claims about a new health risk. This is especially true when health risk research involves new technologies, small numbers of study subjects, and inadequate control groups.

Something akin to this pattern of health risk discovery occurred when mid-twentieth-century American pathologists discovered, promoted, and named new pathological entities, the "in situ" cancers, especially of the breast and cervix, whose definition and meaning straddles the border of risk and disease. Technological innovations such as Pap smears and later screening mammography played important ancillary roles as they led to many women receiving these "precancer" diagnoses. We are still sorting out the significance and implications of these new entities, about which there remains a good deal of uncertainty.

For example, women who received the diagnosis of lobular carcinoma in situ of the breast (LCIS) in the 1950s were often told that they had a kind of menacing early cancer and were frequently encouraged to have "prophylactic" surgery. Later in the century, researchers and clinicians became more aware of the problematic and varied natural history of LCIS. By the end of the century, many clinicians and investigators were thinking of the LCIS diagnosis not so much as an early stage of cancer but as a marker of risk whose magnitude and meaning were uncertain and contested. At the same time, many patients have continued to believe they were suffering from a kind of early cancer and that surgical removal of a small area of LCIS cured them of cancer. Similar problems have been posed by the discovery of the health risks of being a sickle cell disease carrier and of mitral valve prolapse syndrome, which were with time found to be overstated, yet for a brief initial period enjoyed widespread medical credibility.[12] The complex interaction of lay and medical activism, technological change, and other social influences has often led to the rapid — almost instant — construction and naming of health risks, which were, in turn, responded to in ways that would seem, in retrospect, unnecessarily aggressive and/or stigmatizing and whose ontological status would eventually be questioned.

Once discovered and named, health risks need to gain *visibility* among different groups. There is often a protracted time period after the initial discovery or promotion of a health risk during which clinicians, researchers, policy makers, and the larger public become — or fail to become — concerned with the putative links among a particular behavior, an environmental feature, or a biological marker, and ill health. Policy makers might learn a great deal from comparing and contrasting highly visible health risks with those that have not been well accepted and diffused beyond a small group of researchers or advocates, and have had a very long time period between discovery and widespread acceptance and diffusion. For example, why did decades elapse between some clinical and epidemiological observations about tobacco use and lung cancer, and the enlarged visibility of smoking as a major social and public health problem? Historians and others have suggested that diverse interests and values explain this gap: the smoking habits of investigators and opinion leaders, active obfuscation by tobacco growers and cigarette makers, ignorance of and/or resistance to population-based research and its findings, the desire not to blame victims, and fears that the tobacco-cancer association would diminish concern about environmental causes of cancer.[13] Understanding these structured and contingent influences in the extended time period in which some health risks are contested might very well yield insights into new types of health policies aimed at influencing the processes by which health risks gain or do not gain wide public and scientific visibility.

Finally, how is significant *demand* for particular prevention practices and products created? I mean to call attention here to the multifaceted ways that prevention products and practices become used and useable. Policy responses—drug regulation, licensing of screening tests, practice guidelines, etc.—to a new preventive practice are ideally based on critical appraisal of rigorous scientific investigations of the safety and efficacy of particular prevention products and practices. But many products and practices are widely assimilated prior to, or independently of, the creation or assessment of medical evidence about prevention, as was the case with the rapid diffusion of PSA screening in the late 1980s and early 1990s.

Prevention products and practices often develop and diffuse in a piecemeal fashion. They often arise within a context removed from disease prevention, such as the consumer market or behaviors not initially rationalized or understood in terms of their impact on health. For example, many technologies ultimately used as screening tests were not developed for screening or other prevention purposes. Instead they had existing or potential uses for etiologic research (e.g., as a way to determine whether a particular virus might cause a clinical syndrome) as well as diagnosis of disease in clinical practice. So it is often difficult to even locate the moment in time at which certain technologies evolved into screening tests.

The role played by lay advocates in shaping demand for particular prevention practices represents another underappreciated, potential point of policy analysis and intervention.[14] It is also important to consider the ways that different characteristics of target populations have shaped medical and popular demand for prevention practices.

Consider, for example, the different histories of screening mammography for breast cancer and screening chest radiographs and sputum cytology for lung cancer in recent decades. In contrast to screening mammography, there has never been much demand—until very recently—for screening X-rays and sputum cytology to detect lung cancer among smokers. A limited set of studies beginning in the 1950s

suggested that screening did not save lives and that any apparent survival benefit was an illusion created by finding smokers destined to die
of cancer earlier in the course of their disease rather than prolonging
their lives. But these studies had major flaws and were not designed to
test screening against no screening.[15]

Why was there so little demand to improve upon these studies—
and effectively screen smokers for lung cancer—until the 1990s? The
answer cannot reside solely in differences in the effectiveness of lung
cancer and breast cancer screening. Ever since the first randomized
trial of mammography in the 1960s there has been evidence that
screening women under fifty is of limited or no value, but such findings have only fueled controversies and stimulated additional studies.
This is in marked contrast to the absence of any widespread research,
visibility, and agitation for lung cancer screening in response to early
empiric data on the value of such tests. To understand the differences
in demand between mammography and lung cancer screening, we
need to recognize the powerful role of beliefs—for example, smokers
are generally considered to be responsible for their cancer and able to
prevent cancer by quitting, while women who develop breast cancer
are often seen as innocent victims of unknown, random influences.

We might also find new sorts of policy leverage from a closer examination of the many incremental bits of tinkering in clinical practice
that increase medical demand for new risk interventions. Examination of the chronology of developments in screening for hyperlipidemia (such as serum cholesterol tests), for example, makes it clear
that the many small innovations in the way lipid-lowering drugs (such
as the statins) were promoted, marketed, and used had a profound
effect on clinicians' enthusiasm for their use. Before these innovations, clinicians had largely ignored hyperlipidemia in actual practice
despite its acceptance by many researchers and public health workers
as an etiological factor in coronary heart disease (CHD). The change in
clinician practice and beliefs did not simply follow from demonstrations of the efficacy of drug therapy. In the 1980s, the ability to quantitatively measure serum lipids, the elaboration of precise cut-offs for
different types of interventions, and the ability to effectively lower
serum lipid levels with palatable drugs led to a transformation of the
CHD prevention model into something that resembled the diagnosis
and treatment of "real" disease, thus overcoming traditional physician

lack of interest in and suspicion of prevention.[16] The complex and incremental construction of a set of prevention routines, norms, and procedures, as much as or more than novel data about the efficacy of a new class of drugs, thus contributed greatly to important changes in the way this health risk was routinely understood and managed. Policies that encourage or discourage the creation and dissemination of these routines, norms, and procedures can have a profound effect on whether new disease prevention practices are successful or not.

The social history of sex hormones

The recent history of sex hormones (that is, estrogen preparations, sometimes in combination with progesterone, that have most frequently, if misleadingly, been labeled as hormone replacement therapy, or HRT) to prevent chronic disease among postmenopausal women suggests that the social history of health risks can be a tool for evaluating existing disease prevention policies and imagining new ones.[17] In 1941, medical scientists first suggested that estrogen therapy might prevent osteoporosis in postmenopausal women. Additional studies appeared in the 1960s that further supported this proposition. In 1979, the results of a ten-year prospective study on the relationship between estrogen replacement therapy and osteoporosis were published, confirming that estrogen slowed or even reversed bone loss in postmenopausal women.[18] The possible benefits of estrogen in preventing heart disease have perhaps an even longer history, serving to explain the once widely perceived difference in cardiovascular mortality between men and women.

Sex hormone use for osteoporosis and other types of disease prevention have been controversial over this entire period, but analyses of large-scale placebo-controlled randomized clinical trials seemingly resolved the controversy in favor of the skeptics in 2002.[19] The most relevant historical observation about the shaping of demand for sex hormones to prevent disease is that this class of drugs has long had other uses—as contraceptives, to combat infertility, to treat menopausal symptoms, to maintain "femininity"—so that the evaluation of how, when, and among whom these medications were taken for prevention of osteoporosis and heart disease is difficult. For many individuals in different eras and settings, chronic disease prevention was just one of many goals.

Claims about maintaining femininity in the 1960s and 1970s were later eclipsed by others focused on preventing osteoporosis and even later CHD. Watkins described how the rationale for prescribing HRT to menopausal and postmenopausal women has changed over the past four decades.[20] From the 1960s through the mid 1970s, the pharmaceutical industry marketed (and indeed, physicians prescribed) HRT for its putative slowing of the aging process and amelioration of the emotional instability brought on by menopause. However, when studies revealed an association between estrogen use and endometrial cancer, faith in HRT declined and the rationale shifted to the rhetoric of preventing osteoporosis and later cardiovascular disease. MacPherson cited three sequential rationales for HRT use: 1966–75, eternal beauty and femininity; 1975–81, safer symptom-free menopause; 1981–present, escape from chronic disease.[21] These shifting rationales and blurred boundaries have been fundamental in maintaining and even enlarging demand for the drugs prior to the Women's Health Initiative (WHI) results.

Regulators have been hard pressed to evaluate and keep up with these shifts and changes. For example, it was only in 1989 that the FDA officially evaluated and endorsed HRT use for the prevention of osteoporosis. This was years after osteoporosis prevention (and combination therapy with progesterone) reenergized HRT use in the wake of the downturn caused by the discovery that estrogen increased the risk of endometrial cancer.[22]

Many observers have noted that another driving force behind the creation and maintenance of demand for sex hormones has been an alliance between pharmaceutical companies and moral entrepreneurs. Supported by pharmaceutical industry, Robert Wilson's 1966 book *Feminine Forever* is frequently credited with jump-starting estrogen use for menopausal symptoms in the 1960s.[23] Pharmaceutical companies have long recognized that a drug used by every American female over long time periods would create a great market, and they have energetically promoted these drugs through advertising and physician detailing, in addition to sponsoring research, awareness programs, and professional organizations.

Many other investigators and clinicians besides Wilson have received financial support from pharmaceutical companies and pushed for greater HRT use.[24] While I would not claim that the conduct or interpretation of the clinical trials of sex hormones for chronic disease prevention were tainted by the financial support of investigators or by the participation of HRT enthusiasts, such sponsorship or stewardship may very well have affected the content and strength of scientific consensus, as well as kept the use of these drugs on medical and public radar screens.

For example, observational studies have inherent limitations that probably explain the repeated finding of a positive association between HRT and different measures of good health. Unlike randomized trials, subjects are not assigned to treatments. It is difficult in these observational trials to fully adjust for the fact that women who take HRT in the real world generally have healthier attitudes and lifestyles than those who do not take HRT. It is possible, but I know of no supporting evidence, that some sponsors of studies or HRT enthusiasts anticipated and consciously exploited this weakness. A more reasonable but no less troubling inference is that once there was initial evidence for preventive health benefits in observational trials, drug companies could support many different studies, which in turn reported a large number of weakly positive results. (While replication of research results usually strengthens our belief in their reality, repeated studies that share the same inherent biases should not.) Each study was judged on its scientific merits, but the net effect of so many of these weakly positive studies was to increase confidence in the reality of the association and to keep it visible among the general public and medical communities.

At the same time, there have been many persistent, skeptical voices about HRT for chronic disease prevention (as well as treatment of menopausal symptoms) within and outside of medicine. "The increased administration of [HRT]," two feminist critics asserted in 1994, was "yet another form of medical violence against women."[25] Such critics have pointed out the sexist assumptions in constructing menopause as a pathological state: the reductionism inherent in framing menopause as a state of hormone depletion, the cultural myopia and biological determinism in assuming menopausal symptoms are universal, the "heterosexist" assumptions about women's goals and needs, the exploitation of women's fears of aging, and the way that the focus on hormone depletion reflected sexist notions of female frailty and nonnormality.[26]

Despite this opposition, the preventive rationale for HRT use in the 1980s and 1990s became medical and public health received wisdom. There was a good deal of research into medical and lay "noncompliance" as well as educational campaigns by medical associations and public health groups to encourage the preventive use of HRT. But given persistent scientific uncertainty and controversy, the difficulty of weighing small health benefits against health risks like endometrial and breast cancer, and the nuisance and cost of medications, many policy-setting groups ultimately recommended that physicians initiate discussions about HRT use and that women become informed consumers and make decisions for themselves.[27]

The determined efforts of some medical groups, health activists, and pharmaceutical companies to increase compliance notwithstanding, evidence on actual HRT use has generally shown that only a minority of eligible women were ever prescribed these medications, that only a fraction of women prescribed HRT filled these prescriptions, and that only a small fraction actually took the medications for a prolonged period.[28] This pattern of use is important because the putative benefits of these drugs to prevent osteoporosis rested on the assumption that women would maintain their high estrogenic state from menopause through the rest of their lives.

Analysis of data from the WHI suggested no benefit in terms of heart disease, stroke, and dementia and a slight risk of breast cancer in the treatment group, eventually resulting in a premature ending of the trial in July 2002.[29] Along with the coincident reporting of data from other randomized clinical trials, the results of the WHI led to policy statements recommending caution or discontinuation of HRT use to prevent chronic disease. Not surprisingly, this led to a very rapid decline in their use, not only for chronic disease prevention, but also for treatment of menopausal symptoms, since in practice the two purposes were often combined.

This history suggests we need greater public and professional skepticism towards attempts to (1) classify as noncompliant those patients and doctors who do not follow national consensus recommendations and (2) bring uniformity through research and educational campaigns. The physicians and women who were skeptical of HRT use in the 1980s and 1990s may have understood the ability of narrow interests to set the agenda and timing of the prevention landscape. Some skeptics may also have been intuitively repelled by the hubris of conceptualizing women's bodies as needing replacement hormones. Others may have discounted the presumed benefits of HRT because they knew that most people were unlikely to take any medicine daily for the rest of their lives. Certainly these factors contributed to my own reluctance to initiate discussions of the preventive use of HRT with my patients during this period. Many physicians and consumers have also worried about the dangers of new putative risk-reducing drugs because of the fate of other highly promoted medications in the recent past, from the 1950s campaigns to promote DES as a fertility drug to the more recent promotion of phen-fen medications for weight loss as well as the earlier discovery of the risk of endometrial cancer from HRT. A related policy implication, then, is to understand diversity of opinion and practice as a positive factor—and possible source of leverage—in the complex social negotiations over and response to health risks.

We might also more carefully scrutinize those actions of researchers, activists, and clinicians that blur the boundaries between treatment and prevention, and between the relief of symptoms and the promise of continued health. Many women and physicians accepted the risks of sex hormones in treating menopausal symptoms prior to widespread use of these drugs for prevention. This chronology may have contributed to what seems, in retrospect, to have been an overly low threshold for prescribing and using these drugs to prevent chronic disease. This lowered threshold for accepting risk may have resulted from the fact that these drugs were often prescribed for their presumed double effect (treating menopausal symptoms and reducing risk of CHD and osteoporosis).[30]

We might also scrutinize more carefully the increasingly popular resolution of prevention controversies: if the evidence cannot lead to blanket recommendations, decisions should be left to the individual doctor and patient. While this conclusion is perhaps the only way to reach a consensus, it is important to bear in mind that there was a lot of profit to be made by encouraging discussion and shared decision making about hormone use. The mid-1990s consensus that the decision to initiate HRT to prevent osteoporosis and CHD was best made by women themselves, in consultation with their doctors, invited advertising campaigns aimed at prospective users and led to large profits for drug companies. Even a small share of the potential market of all eligible post- or perimenopausal women is very large in absolute terms.

Policy-making groups might be better off concluding that discussions about products and practices for which there is no good evidence of net benefit should not be initiated by medical professionals. Medical silence and inaction, and limits on the promotional activities of self-interested parties, might be the better default position than calling for shared decision making. Why should clinical uncertainty automatically trigger a policy reflex to "let the patient decide," especially when one of the options is a preventive medication with possible serious side effects or a screening test that can lead to the harms of unnecessary treatment? If expert policy groups cannot come to an informed judgment, why expect the average American to exercise judgment by default?

The fact that pharmaceutical companies and other groups can potentially manage the flow of scientific data by the timing and intensity of funding, by defining the questions they are willing to fund, and by taking advantage of or manipulating the inherent limitations of studies suggests the need for some oversight over how health risks are *discovered* and made *visible*. A similar policy response also follows from the fact that much of the *demand* for HRT use was generated by women's groups and health care workers who genuinely wanted to make women live longer and healthier lives and who felt that they were redressing a historical neglect of older women's health issues. These groups and individuals drew credibility and power from the resonance of this message throughout the medical and lay community, as well as its obvious appeal to pharmaceutical concerns. Thus we need some counterweight to the power and influence of moral entrepreneurs with a financial or professional stake in the success of particular health risks and disease prevention practices. Good intentions do not immunize them from advocating bad policies. The moral and material synergy among these different actors requires careful analysis and a strategic response.

At the same time, other individuals and groups were marginalized in the clinical and policy response to the putative health risks posed by "hormone deficiency." Critical commentary on the dangers of medicalizing normal aging and the hegemony, narrow perspective, economic bias, and sexism of medical and pharmaceutical promoters of HRT largely occurred on different turf from the medical controversy over efficacy and risk that played out in medical journals and consensus conferences.

Taken together, these historical observations represent an argument for policy mechanisms that make visible and better incorporate the perspectives of the many social critics who have pointed out the limitations in how knowledge of health risks is generated, legitimated, and used as the basis for action. One response is to develop or encourage new activist lay constituencies that advocate caution and point out the dangers of iatrogenic harm and medical hubris. We have not tapped the potential of the unorganized but numerous individuals who are unhappily medicalized, suffer side effects of screening or prevention practices, and pay the economic costs of expensive but useless or marginally beneficial prevention practices. These voices ought to be heard more clearly in prevention debates and might constitute a force with wide societal credibility. Adding these voices to policy-making processes would allow simultaneous consideration of the apples and oranges of cultural criticism and medical data. For example, such groups might have weighed the advantages and disadvantages of medicalizing menopause, conceptualizing women's bodies as hormone deficient, or viewing osteoporosis as a female disease at the same time that there was a critical appraisal of medical and epidemiological data.

This new kind of prevention oversight body might work under the auspices of a prestigious scientific body like the Institute of Medicine. A dose of realism is needed here, however. Policy change will occur only if the rationale is made visible and compelling to actors in the political process—and there has been little societal or medical awareness of the need for such upstream prevention policy interventions.

Lastly, the social history of HRT use in American society reminds us that other approaches to improving the health of the elderly have been neglected by the way the problem was conceptualized and labeled in the *discovery* stage. Conceptualizing and labeling osteoporosis as a latent condition emanating from hormonal loss in menopause, to be cured by pills strategically labeled as "hormone replacements," narrowed policy options. A self-evident consequence has been the myopic lack of interest in male bone weakness. The focus on maintaining bone density through drugs also shifted attention away from the problem of older women breaking hips or knees, whether from "thin" bones, losing their balance or ability to walk, or neglecting their diet or exercise. More generally, the construction of these risks as individual medical problems to be solved by drugs discouraged a population approach. Defining the policy debate as weighing evidence about HRT use and demineralization, for example, obscured the formulation of the problem as one of injury prevention. Compared to the considerable societal angst over HRT use, there has been little interest in a population approach to injury prevention through better housing, reduced poverty, less social isolation, and greater social services.

Conclusions

I have suggested that we need new sorts of oversight, debate, and influence over how risks are discovered, promoted, and made objects of disease prevention. We might begin with new types of regulatory bodies with purview over publically financed health research, which would more closely scrutinize the research and development of screening technologies that have no proven means of effective treatment or evasion (for example, some screening tests for genetic risk of common diseases, such as Alzheimer's).[31]

Just raising the issue of constraining research necessarily invites a broad debate. The policy response to this problem is complex, in part because unconstrained scientific inquiry, technological innovation, and market freedom are highly valued. It is also difficult to know what kinds of knowledge will eventually prove useful. On the other hand, the sheer magnitude of the health risks that can be forged from associations between genetic and other health outcomes and their potential for evidence-free diffusion into clinical practice and consumer use forces us to ask whether certain types of health risk research need regulation at the early stages of their development. This complex political, ethical, and scientific debate is unavoidable because different individuals and groups stand to gain or lose depending on which risks and practices are accepted. Historical analysis can contribute to this debate by identifying developments that were not inevitable and might have been subject to more explicit debate and policy intervention.

Existing forms of practice regulation, such as our short-sighted regulatory focus on new drugs with limited indications, may need to be reevaluated. We need to do a better job of monitoring and regulating the efficacy and safety of prevention technologies, drugs, and practices in the shifting and ambiguous contexts in which they are actually used. We may want to examine and regulate tests and drugs whose context of use has shifted (not merely when manufacturers request a change in product indication and labeling) as if they were entirely new tests and drugs.

We might also want to better scrutinize how health risks are promoted and publicized. Commercial sponsorship of research may need greater checks than our current protections, such as disclosure of funding and peer review in scientific publications. I have suggested that our public health goals might be expanded to include educational campaigns intended to influence medical and consumer risk–related attitudes and behaviors, such as those aimed at recognizing and preventing medicalization and iatrogenesis as much as putative health risks.[32]

Other relatively unexplored policy responses might be considered. Can we better integrate the cultural and political critique often passionately advanced by lay activists with the processes and outcomes of evidence-based scientific review? Can we find better ways to empower and make visible the interests of the many individuals who are affected by the overselling of health risks because of increased cost and inconvenience, iatrogenic mishaps, or unwelcome messages about their health and lifestyle choices? While these and other questions raised by situating health risks in their social and historical context are difficult to answer, we have ample reasons to begin asking them.

10

Epilogue: The risk system

We have often hastily and with hubris identified new health risks and then devised and diffused risk-reducing interventions before knowing whether they were safe and efficacious in the long run. The self-evident logic and fear-controlling appeal of risk reduction has often trumped caution. Even voicing skepticism can seem shrill and insensitive given the promise to ward off disease and death. The emotion-laden controversy that not surprisingly surrounds many risk-related practices is all the more reason to analyze them objectively and with some detachment.

So I want to conclude by emphasizing that linking different lay, clinical, and public health ideas and practices in the U.S. and other economically advanced societies—and as I pointed out in chapter 8, globally as well—is a *risk system*. In this epilogue, I describe some important components of this system and the logic that binds them into something larger than the sum of its parts. I will sketch a general picture of the system and then explore (1) the problematic "states of risk" that often create demand for more interventions, (2) the self-fulfilling and self-reinforcing features of many risk systems, (3) the (often ironic) interconnectedness of risk interventions, (4) the centrality of trust, and (5) some clinical and policy implications.

The risk system

Reducing risk is no longer a means to health but often its very definition. To comply with screening protocols, have acceptable numbers on blood tests or images on scans, and engage in behaviors believed to lower risk, is—despite the evident circularity—to be healthy.

The biomedical pursuit of earlier points in the natural history of disease and the increasing intensity of medical interventions propel medical and lay people towards this risk-centered conception of ill health and even more risk interventions. Risk is more than just knowledge of probabilistic associations. People often live a life at risk, associated with fear, loss of control, and the work of self-surveillance and other risk-reducing behaviors. Increasingly, this risk state is part of, or follows, a diagnosis of chronic disease.

Risk interventions are increasingly taken up because they putatively reduce the risk of other interventions, another multiplier effect. Fear and restoration of control drive the uptake and diffusion of both scientifically validated and evidence-challenged interventions.

Risk-reducing products and practices also bring profits to manufacturers, clinicians, and others. These financial rewards are sustained by the easily expanded demand for many risk interventions, which can involve entire populations for most of their life spans. Some successful risk-reducing ideas and practices operate similar to what economists call *rents*. Tolls are collected from the stable traffic of consumers and patients utilizing products and practices that have monopoly-like status from patents and mandates from expert advisory boards, and whose costs are often hidden at point of purchase by third-party arrangements.

One sweet spot for reaping market rewards is the junction of common symptoms and risk reduction. A good example is the obstructive sleep apnea diagnosis and the interventions the diagnosis triggers. People go to high-tech sleep laboratories because of interrupted sleep and daytime fatigue. Often their bed partners notice bouts of nonbreathing and excessive snoring. The objective high-tech fee-generating evaluation may lead to a diagnosis of sleep apnea, a converged disease-risk state. On the one hand, sleep apnea causes chronic symptoms, both in the quality of sleep and its effects on daytime function. But sleep apnea is also a risk state, because it is associated with serious long-term risks, such as restrictive lung disease and heart failure that may follow from chronic inadequate oxygenation. Both symptoms and risk are often treated by continuous positive airway pressure (CPAP). The intervention promises less snoring and better daytime function as well as reduced risk of chronic lung and heart disease and sudden death.

Observers estimate that obstructive sleep apnea prevalence in the U.S. is in the tens of millions.[1] While there is solid evidence linking severe apnea to serious health problems, there is a dearth of good data on the long-term efficacy and safety of interventions for people with mild problems, whose decisions for evaluation and intervention may be heavily influenced by the promise to reduce the long-term risks of untreated sleep apnea. Yet there has been both massive diffusion of both the risk/disease state, i.e. the sleep apnea diagnosis, and the risk intervention, CPAP.[2]

Crucial to the diffusion and stability of many well-established risk systems is an experienced risk state whose work and psychological dimensions create their own demand for intervention. Prostatic specific antigen (PSA) screening, for example, often leads to a diagnosis of good-prognosis cancer that has such a low and uncertain chance of serious harm that it can be understood as an embodied state of risk. It is often not clear whether to intervene with surgery or radiation or do the intense surveillance that constitutes "watchful waiting." For many clinicians and patients, the latter option results in a risk state that is actively experienced. Some patients perceive the sword of Damocles hovering continuously over their heads. Uncertainty, ambiguity, and ambivalence follow from leaving a potentially deadly but curable cancer in their bodies. Their doctors may recommend a slew of tests and surveillance routines that often trigger radical treatments by signaling disease progression and/or create an experience so profoundly unsettling and full of work that patients and doctors often end up opting for a more radical solution to be done with it.

The risk system also works by practices that transform epidemiological realities and perceptions in directions that further sustain their use. As a result of prostate cancer screening, we have a greatly enlarged population of people who are diagnosed with cancer and who live long cancer-free lives. The individuals themselves and others often believe their lives have been saved by screening and invasive treatment. In addition, many of these individuals become advocates for the entire early detection paradigm and sustain its use by recruiting others and influencing funding and other policies.

Modern cancer survivorship, explored in chapter 7, is perhaps the largest example of a converged disease-risk system. Early detection and screening, new precancerous diagnoses, lowered pathological thresholds, and other factors have contributed to the rapid growth in the number of cancer survivors. Knowledge of lifetime risks associated with cancer and its treatments, the intensity and multiple modalities of treatment, and the increasingly long life span after initial treatment have led to greatly expanded concern, self-surveillance, and interventions for cancer survivors. Current estimates of American cancer survivors are twelve million people. Given that many more may harbor cancerous cells in their bodies or have genetic evidence of cancer risk, it is plausible that there might be a doubling or tripling or more of cancer survivors in the next decades, especially as more sensitive probes are developed and new risks identified. Given the morbidity of some risk interventions, and the work and cost of some cancer-surviving routines and practices, this could be a dystopian future, especially if this massive expansion is not accompanied by a significant reduction in cancer mortality and morbidity.

Some thoughtful critics within medicine have dealt with the expansion of cancer diagnoses as an overdiagnosis problem, but this label falls short of capturing the entire phenomenon and its challenges.[3] Overdiagnosis implies that the diagnosis is a mistake. But not only is overdiagnosis only reliably understood from an aggregate perspective, the label does not capture the positive meaning many people find in the career or identity of being a survivor.

Emerging states of risk

One emerging risk system involves people at risk for Alzheimer's disease (AD). We do not know the cause or causes of AD, or exactly what the disease is at the level of the brain, or whether it is a brain disease exclusively, or a single disease or many. Despite or perhaps because of all that we do not know, many efforts have been and are being made to prevent the disease or alter its course once started. In recent years, we have had largely unsuccessful drug interventions for people with symptomatic AD, targeting the plaques and tangles associated with the disease, restoring acetylcholine levels, and other interventions aimed at putative mechanisms or pathways.

One response to this frustrating failure has been to shift intervention to presumed earlier stages in the disease's natural history, first to mild and moderate disease, and more recently to asymptomatic people at presumed high risk of the disease. For example, there are ongoing trials in which people at high risk of AD on the basis of genetic tests and biomarkers are given antibodies to neurofibrillary tangles.[4] Underlying this shift to treating risk are assumptions about the high likelihood of progression to declining mental status among those at risk and the causative role played by tangles or other mechanisms.

Many people have worried about the negative psychological impact of creating a class of people who are "at risk for Alzheimer's disease," a side effect of these trials and the diffusion of knowledge about this risk state. How do we balance the potential upsides of doing this research with the potential fear and anxiety that might follow from being identified and labeled as at high risk of the disease?

A major pharmaceutical company conducting one of these AD prevention trials invited me to participate in a group charged with exploring this question and other ethical, legal, and social dimensions of these trials. I declined the invitation because I did not want to have, or even create the impression of having, a financial conflict of interest (and thus compromised objectivity) by accepting payments by the sponsoring drug company. I also feared that the group, whatever the intentions of its members, would ultimately serve to smooth out the bumps and provide moral cover ("look, we thought about these issues") for a research and marketing commitment already launched.

But I would have liked to have been a fly on the wall during these discussions and to have had a chance to express my concern that these trials can contribute to a *risk system* that may make difficult future evidence-based challenges to the use of biomarkers to define risk states and of preventive drugs. The failure to progress to AD may be experienced by some participants in and out of the trial as evidence that risk interventions work. Being identified as "high risk" may have more systemic consequences than causing anxiety and fear in some people. At an aggregate level, it may catalyze, as has happened with the embodied HPV risk state and among people living with screening-detected prostate cancer, more demand for interventions—such as the drugs used in these trials or other screening or preventative maneuvers—that reduce or manage the risk state itself. The expanded class of people at risk who may do work (e.g., participate in AD screening and surveillance, take preventive medications, and/or make lifestyle changes) and have somatic evidence (biomarkers) of risk, may converge with the mass of AD patients (with its already wide spectrum) and the disease advocates (in the case of AD, usually family members, who themselves are or may believe they are at high risk) into a large pool for further advocacy for early intervention.

While clinical research in AD is extremely important, the potential negative impacts of expanding the diagnosis' catchment area should not be ignored. Even limited diffusion of AD prevention can contribute to the visibility and plausibility of AD risk states, creating fear and desperation, leading to the use of experimental drugs and practices outside of trials. Once a new risk system has been stabilized, it can be resistant to evidence-based challenge. Before allowing risk systems to stabilize, we need disinterested evaluation and regulation of the practices that create them.[5]

Perceptions of efficacy and looping effects

Things we know or think we know about the probabilities of different outcomes and risk interventions shape individual decisions and practices. And the resulting behavior change, in aggregate, can influence how researchers, clinicians, patients, and consumers perceive the plausibility of risks and the efficacy of interventions, leading to more behavior change. They constitute looping effects.[6]

In 2007, when former New York City mayor Rudy Giuliani was an aspiring Republican presidential candidate, he would often mention his own experience as a prostate cancer survivor as evidence of the superiority of the American "free market" health care system over those of countries that had socialized medical care. Giuliani claimed that "my chance of success here in America is just much better than anyplace else in the world . . . The chance of a man surviving prostate cancer in the United States is somewhere, when I was doing it, 82 percent,

84 percent. It's probably over 90 percent now. In socialized medicine countries, it's—some of them can be less than 50 percent, and none of them like the United States . . . The chances of surviving [breast cancer] in the United States for a woman are much greater than in France, or in England, or in Canada, or in Cuba, where Michael Moore would like us all to go for health care."[7]

Giuliani was not making up these statistics. In fact, the five-year survival rate for prostate cancer as reported by the National Cancer Institute's SEER system (a highly respected survey of cancer incidence, mortality, and other indicators) was an astounding 99 percent by 2007.[8] Survival rates in the other countries "with socialized medicine" were less good. But Giuliani was wrong in inferring that his "chance of success" was any better in the U.S. than anywhere else. What matters to most us is whether we live longer or better. The five-year survival rates in the U.S. approach 100 percent because prostate cancer mortality has remained within a relatively narrow range during recent decades, while cancer diagnoses have increased tremendously.[9] Survival rates, or their inverse, case-fatality rates, are ratios of numbers of people diagnosed to numbers dying, and they necessarily increase if the death rate remains relatively stable and the numbers of diagnosed increase. With estimates that 1 in 6 American men receiving a diagnosis of prostate cancer in their lifetime, the still high but not dramatically changing death rate from prostate cancer of approximately 30,000 American men a year necessarily means we have a very high survival rate.

Giuliani's perceptions are central to the reflexive, self-reinforcing system that supports beliefs in the efficacy of many risk interventions like PSA screening. People take up risk interventions, resulting in changes in survival statistics, perceptions of a disease's severity, and the efficacy of those same interventions. This leads to more use of interventions, and more changes in perceptions of the target disease and the efficacy of interventions.

These looping effects help explain why some risk interventions become mass phenomena in short periods of time and seem resistant to dislodging by evidence questioning their efficacy and safety. While a few voices in the late 1980s and early 1990s raised ethical questions about the mass diffusion of PSA testing before there were randomized clinical trials assessing its efficacy and safety, most physicians at that time felt that using a technology that could detect cancer "early" and lead to treatment when it was still curable was the only defensible course of action. Results from clinical trials of PSA screening were not available until the late 2000s. They showed either no mortality impact from PSA screening or a small impact at the questionable cost of surgical and other harm to many men who did not benefit. But after over two decades of PSA screening, an entire stable system of action and perception was in place, so the results from these clinical trials have had little impact on practice. Moreover, the likelihood of ever knowing whether there are objective health benefits to mass risk interventions like PSA screening has been seriously diminished because practices have diffused so widely that there are too many people getting screened in the "usual care" control arms of large-scale screening experiments to really know if a "no effect" result is real or not.[10]

One risk intervention leads to another: Rational entry but often no exit

I am a four-year-old kindergartner. My task is to draw my family, and my teacher says to begin by making a border. My first lines are crooked, so I try to straighten them by making them thicker. More crookedness ensues, more widening, and soon there is no space to draw anyone or anything. This outcome—and my sense of inadequacy—reminds me of some of our compensatory reactions to other imperfect practices in risk-centered medicine today, such as the way practices are invented, introduced, and diffused because they reduce the harm and cost of other risk interventions. Like my uneven four-year-old hand, one compensation creates the need for another. I fear that soon there may be little space, that is money, attention span, and trust, for whatever it is we wanted to accomplish in the first place.

In a documentary film that captures patient decision making about reconstructive surgery after breast cancer, the central person featured is a plastic surgeon with a wry sense of humor and offbeat bedside manner. She repeatedly discusses the option of removing not just the breast with cancer but the unaffected one, followed by bilateral breast reconstruction. This surgeon never promises better survival. Instead, she repeatedly says that the removal of both breasts, in addition to representing an opportunity to get a desired cosmetic effect, will cure women of their need for mammograms.[11] In other words, the work done by this radical intervention is to reduce the trouble of another risk intervention.

Sociologists have argued that the risks associated with technology, and the technological responses to those risks, which often carry their own uncertainties and provoke other responses, are characteristic features of advanced, modern societies. The way one health risk evokes another is a characteristic of our *risk society*. Beck, Giddens, and other modern risk theorists make far-reaching observations about risk and its central role in defining what is modern, postmodern, or secondarily modern about today's industrialized societies. Societies are wracked by problems of uncertainty, often arising out of science and technology, and face often invisible threats that do not respect nation-state borders, such as climate change or fallout from nuclear accidents. According to Beck and colleagues, "this 'meta-change' of modern society results from a critical mass of unintended side-effects. By unintended side-effects—or more precisely, effects that were originally intended to be more narrow in their scope than they turned out to be—we mean the host of consequences resulting from the boundary-shattering force of market expansion, legal universalism and technical revolution."[12]

Many modern health risk interventions, with origins in market expansion and technological change, have unintended and unanticipated far-reaching effects.[13] What is perhaps characteristic of health risks is that the "host of consequences" is mediated not only by their physical and objective impacts on bodies, but also by the way risk knowledge is itself unsettling, leading to actions and states of mind that create other problems.

Risk interventions, however, can and often do have very real bodily impacts, especially in the context of chronic disease. A close friend was put on an antiestrogen after a lumpectomy for locally invasive breast cancer. This medication is believed to lower the risk of cancer recurrence.[14] After a short period on the medicine, my friend developed hot flashes. Her oncologist then prescribed an antidepressant, not for any mood or affect disorder, but because the medication was believed to be efficacious against this side effect. After finishing her course of preventative treatment with the antiestrogen, my friend tried to stop taking the antidepressant but each time she experienced hot flashes, irritability, and sleep disturbance. These symptoms were hard to distinguish from depression, but there was no reason to diagnose depression in my friend. She never appeared to be suffering an affect disorder of any kind, just side effects from another risk intervention. Nevertheless, the intervention had seemingly changed something in the body, creating a need to continue taking it.

We often have very limited knowledge of the long-term safety and efficacy of interventions, whether targeting risk, ameliorating symptoms, or curing disease. Another close friend had suffered for decades with pain and hematological and joint problems that did not line up very well with any single disease category. His doctors cautiously improvised with different treatments, and my friend was largely able to function and live a full, active life. Decades later he developed leukemia. My friend and his doctors suspect that one of the drugs that helped stabilize his pain and joint disease was partly or wholly responsible for this new, aggressive cancer.

The intensity of our medical interventions and their very success in improving function and warding off death have led us to the complex reality where the longer-term risks of interventions are becoming more apparent and consequential. Even when the longer-term risks of interventions are known, we often do not have enough precise information about their benefits and dangers to be confident in the wisdom of clinical decisions at the time they are made. Clinicians, patients, and their loved ones may experience regret and confusion over past decisions, but who is to say whether these decisions were not the right ones given what was known and knowable at the time they were made?

In the case of my friend, these uncertainties were never ignored. He and his doctor calculated benefits and risks together and were aware of what was known and not known. Few of us would argue that we should treat severe joint pain or other serious medical problems only with interventions for which we have solid evidence of long-term efficacy and safety. In many situations, taking a drug or consenting to some procedure for which there is less-than-ideal evidence of net long-term benefit makes more sense than inaction or alternatives that carry their own risks and uncertainties. Moreover, in some moments of crisis, like the early years of the AIDS epidemic, many of us were in favor of relaxing standards of drug and technology assessment and regulation in order to get drugs of unknown benefit to often desperate patients who wanted them and had little to lose.[15]

But we need to account for the impact of such practices in aggregate, how they interact, and the resulting system that is not simply the sum of the parts. Here is where we need more level-headed and detached analysis. For example, the immune-modulating medicine for arthritis implicated in my friend's cancer is directly advertised to consumers in television and print advertisements. The cancer risk of this medicine is mentioned only within a long list of many other serious complications, all of which, the television advertisement says, "have occurred."[16] The mass selling of a drug with very narrow approved indications, using slick advertisements that lump different dangers in language that obfuscates dangers is irresponsible. Scientific caution that association does not mean causality is not a reason to obscure possible dangers. This advertisement and the aggressive selling of similar interventions minimize our considerable uncertainty about long-term benefits and risks and invites overtreatment and use in nonindicated situations. This creation and exploitation of demand deserves more and tighter regulation, as I argued in the previous chapter.

Advances in medical knowledge and therapeutics have created a tragic situation in the classical sense that the seeds of bad outcomes are intrinsic, foreordained. They follow from what we want: powerful interventions that relieve pain, cure cancer, etc. But the dilemmas, regrets, and uncertainties that sometimes follow are not just problems for affected individuals. They are leading indicators of larger societal and medical problems. I call special attention to our ignorance of the long-term safety and efficacy of health risk interventions because they are often mass interventions whose effects may take decades to reliably measure. Yet the appeal of prevention and the logic of reducing risk have often led to their rapid and widespread diffusion.

Patients and their clinicians typically enter the risk system together, mostly with their eyes open, often with similar motivations, hopes, and fears. There is no medical conspiracy, nor are even the most controversial ideas and actions simply reducible to a false consciousness, conflict of interest, or other nefarious influences. I avail myself of some risk interventions (two screening colonoscopies), and bury my head in the sand for others. I continuously remind my primary care doctor to not check the PSA box when my blood is drawn for other reasons, but even this might change as I age and review new evidence or simply tire of resisting. Some individuals are helped by medical risk interventions, some hurt, while most are unaffected. But evaluating the risk system, the logic and aggregate inputs and impacts of these linked ideas and practices, is not solely an individual matter, and presents different challenges and responses from a societal perspective.

I would not second-guess the decision of someone with breast cancer who opts for surgery to remove the unaffected breast, even as I am very concerned about the rapid increase in contralateral prophylactic mastectomies across all stages of disease in recent years (see chapter 2). At the societal level, we need to critically examine whether screening programs and other practices constitute a self-reinforcing system, driving fear of cancer as well as an overestimation of the efficacy of interventions. While understanding the societal-level dynamics can be helpful to an individual contemplating a difficult decision, that person is often too far out on a limb to think about retracing his or her steps. In addition, individuals necessarily weigh odds of help and harm from a very different perspective than a policy maker deciding what is best for a population.[17]

The massive explosion of knowledge of gene-disease correlations and biomarkers and the market rewards of mass interventions, among other influences, make the challenge of risk interventions a pressing concern. There is no obvious exit from this system, and few of us would want to retreat from the considerable benefits and promise of much of modern medicine. But piecemeal attention and response have not been sufficient, and understanding the larger social context of particular practices can suggest other ways to maneuver within the risk system.

Centrality of trust

A decision to get screened for disease or take a pill to reduce risk depends on trust in the workings of biomedical science much more than in the past. Practitioners, patients, and consumers value and depend on the most objective and unbiased evidence from rigorous clinical and public health experiments. But the details of knowledge production and interpretation are exceedingly complex and the factors shaping results are only partially visible in scientific reports. Moreover, almost no risk reduction has any direct and perceivable impact on the body, so there is no basis for the individual patient or consumer to reliably monitor an effect based on bodily reactions. As a result, practitioners, patients, and consumers are persuaded to act only if they trust the professionals and institutions that produce and frame the implications of the evidence. They need to feel confident in the smooth workings of the gears and levers of the epidemiological and biomedical machinery that makes and stabilizes the linkages between risk interventions and desired health outcomes. Although central to the operating of the risk system, this trust is often unstable and easily undermined.

Few experts, let alone clinicians and patients/consumers, have the time and expertise to investigate every study and inquire about the reliability and credibility of investigators and their methods. Instead, experts and laypeople usually act on the basis of a more global trust in the actors, institutions, and knowledge-making machinery that make and certify the meaning of the evidence. This was a corollary point to my historical observation in chapter 3 that the multiple roles played by the randomized controlled trial—as truth-making machinery and as means for persuading people to buy and use practices and products—emerged at the same moment. One role is not reducible to the other. Insofar as we are explaining why individuals choose to do some risk interventions and not others, there may be no meaningful boundary between the role played by the perceived truth value of particular bits of evidence and the credibility of those people and institutions who make and evaluate evidence.

The trust underlying the use of particular products and practices is all too easily constructed and eroded. I evoked earlier an "easy come, easy go" phenomenon in which the social efficacy of a risk intervention, built on trust in linkages between a product or practice and a health outcome, was rapidly built up and just as quickly dissipated, for example the rapid rise and sudden fall of Vioxx or the market failure of Lyme disease vaccines following upon initial high enthusiasm from lay and medical people.

I often invite a prominent infectious disease physician and vocal opponent of vaccine skeptics to talk to one of my undergraduate classes. My students learn a lot from my colleague's convincing take-down of spurious associations between vaccines and autism and claims that taking multiple vaccines simultaneously is dangerous to children. But I worry that his "take no prisoners" dismissal of vaccine skepticism and exclusive focus on bad theories and shaky evidence does not give enough attention to the complicated dynamics between laypeople and scientific expertise that undergirds trust in the vaccine enterprise. Parents' near total compliance with standard vaccine recommendations is unprecedented in clinical medicine and public health. This compliance works because of an unusually high degree of trust in public health authorities' advisories and belief in their overall credibility.

One potential source of mistrust and the proclivity to accept alternative theories are those practices of vaccine producers and promoters that invite doubts about whether they are unbiased and working for the public good. Staunch defenders of the vaccine enterprise can be myopically focused on scientific evidence and harms to children while they ignore the practices that erode trust. Trust can be damaged when the vaccine manufacturers seek profits by aggressively working to make marginal vaccines part of the canon of required ones (by, say, lobbying state legislatures) or set exorbitant prices for vaccines that preclude their use in markets that need but cannot afford them.[18] Or when manufacturers market vaccines with the same ethos and techniques used to sell toothpaste and other consumer products.[19]

Because of the important role this easily damaged trust plays in the risk system, I disagreed with this same colleague's criticisms of the Centers for Disease Control and Prevention's Advisory Committee on Immunization Practices' weak and hedged recommendations for the Lyme disease vaccine (see chapter 5). I believe the committee correctly understood that relevant considerations in their deliberations were factors unrelated to evidence from clinical trials, but shaped the trust various stakeholders have in the vaccine enterprise. In addition to evidence of safety and efficacy, this regulatory committee at least wrestled with issues such as whether the vaccine reduced the risk of a minor or serious health problem, was appealing because of objective health benefits or the reassurance it provided to people afraid of their environments, and was likely to be used by people who most benefited or by other groups.[20]

For similar reasons, I have an ongoing, if minor, disagreement with one of my former students who is very concerned with the threats to the overall workings of the vaccine enterprise by parents and pediatricians who negotiate alternative schedules for administering childhood vaccines. Her concerns are legitimate, as alternative schedules might lead to less individual protection and reduced herd immunity and to a creeping weakening of the authority of regulatory bodies to influence practice. But I have an additional concern, motivated by the central role of trust in the vaccine enterprise. Perhaps some parents' desire to create their own, more spread out, schedule of vaccinations is an acceptable (in terms of potential damage to individual and herd immunity) cost for giving them an outlet for their ambivalence about the validity and wisdom of expert opinion and their own obedience to central authority. Looked at this way, alternative schedules for childhood vaccines might work as a relief or overflow valve for a trust system that demands a lot from parents. Especially because it involves children, "take it or leave it" recommendations may exacerbate anxieties about our always limited ability to know the best course of action. From the perspective of how trust operates within a risk system, it may be wise to let a few alternative flowers bloom.

Precautionary principles

When I imagine the far-reaching implications of understanding much of modern medicine and health-related consumer practice as a *risk system*, I think about the following Yiddish joke:

A young man boarded a train bound for Odessa and sat down next to a prosperous-looking passenger. "Can you tell me the time, sir?" the young man asked. The stranger glanced at him contemptuously. "Drop dead!" he answered. "What the devil is wrong with you!" the young man exploded indignantly. "I ask you as a gentleman and you answer so rudely. What is the problem?" The other passenger made as if to ignore him, then sighing, he turned and said: "All right, I'll tell you.

First you ask a question and I am supposed to answer, yes? So I tell you the time. Then you start up with discussion about the weather, about politics, about the war, about business—soon we discover we are both Jews. So what happens? I live in Odessa and you are a stranger there so I must extend Jewish hospitality and invite you to my home. You meet Sophie, my beautiful daughter, and after a few more visits you both fall in love. Finally, you ask my blessing so that you and Sophie can get married. So why not avoid this big megillah? I can tell you right now, young man, that I positively refuse to let my daughter marry anyone who cannot even afford a watch."[21]

What does this have to do with risk? I often feel that an appropriate societal response to the *risk system* is to act like this curmudgeonly father who refuses to talk, trying to protect the anticipated harms to the marriage prospects for his beautiful daughter. Instead of all the contingent steps to marriage, I am imagining stopping or limiting some of the early stages of the risk system, before practices are stabilized and become resistant to challenge by evidence. But the humor in this tale comes from the difficulty and absurdity of refusing to talk or exchange information in the present because of what it might mean— through a series of anticipated but ultimately unpredictable middle steps—way down the line. Despite this problem, let me cautiously reiterate and expand upon the point I made in the previous chapter, generalized slightly into some precautionary principles or at least a precautionary attitude about health risk knowledge creation and practice diffusion.[22]

The scope of these principles and this skepticism is not just risk-related knowledge and practice as it impacts the asymptomatic would-be patient recruited into a new diagnosis, but patients with bona fide chronic disease. The same critical attention that sociologists and policy makers have paid to medicalizing the previously healthy might profitably be directed towards the growing class of people experiencing a convergence of risk and disease.

The mass diffusion of prostate cancer screening prior to results from randomized clinical trials is evidence of why we need precautionary principles. For new screening or other preventive practices that have the potential to rapidly diffuse and transform our beliefs about and responses to the target condition, we should understand the "randomize the first patient" principle—limiting practice change to careful experiments—as an ethical, not merely scientific, one.[23] We need to prevent harm, not just bad biomedical science.

In the previous chapter, I cautiously entered into the territory of "upstream" policy interventions as well as attitudinal change focused on regulating the creation and diffusion of some risk knowledge. I do not claim to have a clear idea of how this would work in practice and remain uneasy about controls on knowledge production per se. But at the same time the pressures to act downstream—at the bedside, office, or online store—are often too powerful for the individual patient, consumer, or health care worker to resist. Empowering such individuals and informed discussion of available medical options are an important, though not sufficient, response by itself.

Peggy Orenstein, a prominent journalist, had a lumpectomy and radiation for breast cancer. The cancer had been picked up by a baseline mammography at age thirty-five, in anticipation of yearly screening starting at age forty. The experience made her a vocal and visible advocate for screening mammography, and she wrote about her experiences for the New York Times. But over the intervening years, her attitude changed, and she became much more skeptical of the early detection and radical treatment paradigm in breast cancer. Her old and new selves were brought into clear contrast when she had a local recurrence of her breast cancer. She was faced with the choice of mastectomy in the affected breast, or a more radical option, taken by an increasing number of women: complete removal of the unaffected as well as the affected breast (contralateral prophylactic mastectomy). Orenstein ultimately decided not to join the growing numbers of women opting for contralateral prophylactic mastectomy in situations like her own, aka "doing everything" to save herself from a future breast cancer death. Orenstein wrote in another New York Times article years later: "What did doing 'everything' mean, anyway? There are days when I skip sunscreen. I don't exercise as much as I should. I haven't given up aged Gouda despite my latest cholesterol count; I don't get enough calcium. And, oh, yeah, my house is six blocks from a fault line. Is living with a certain amount of breast-cancer risk really so different? I decided to take my doctor's advice, to do only what had to be done."[24]

Orenstein struggled but came to the conclusion that she did not need to "do everything" to prevent a feared outcome. Such individual decisions are helped by good data and interpretation from experts who have no actual or perceived conflict of interest. But I remain concerned that we need more than individual responses to the challenges posed by the *risk system*. We may also need some way of making it more difficult to launch and widely diffuse untested practices and products in the first place. This is especially true for risk ideas and interventions that have the potential to transform their target disease, to radically change the makeup of people who are labeled with the risk or disease, and to create the conditions for rapid self-reinforcing diffusion and resistance to future evidence-based challenge. In these situations, we may need some upstream *prevention of prevention*.

In some situations an effective policy response to the excesses of the risk system may be to exploit the social efficacy of less harmful interventions. In the 1960s, aspirin use in children for viral infections was associated with liver and brain damage. Public health authorities' warnings of the dangers of aspirin use in children, what came to be known as Reye's syndrome, were not in themselves sufficient to rapidly change behavior. What was crucial was the promotion of an alternative product with the same or similar social and scientific efficacy, an effective substitute that parents could give their children with fever, cough, and discomfort. This came in the form of the mass marketing of acetaminophen (Tylenol).[25]

More disease, less risk

I have long been part of the chorus of medical critics who have urged that clinical care and medical education be more focused on the individual and less on his or her disease. I have been particularly vocal about caring for people whose suffering has no agreed-upon mechanism or disease name.[26] So there is some irony that one implication of the *risk system* is to rebalance clinical and public health practices in a more disease-oriented direction: more focus on alleviating symptoms and modifying active disease processes, less on preventing disease or future complications of disease; or at least greater skepticism and a "show me the evidence" response about new risks and risk interventions.[27]

One place where the border between disease and risk might be more closely monitored is in the leeway we allow clinicians and patients to make decisions based on considerations of idiosyncrasy and/or an individual's desperate circumstances. A patient with a chronic illness might learn from trying different treatments that a particular medicine, despite what is known from clinical trials, gives relief from pain much better than cheaper alternatives that are supposed to work on average in the same or similar ways. In this situation, it makes sense to pay attention to the individual's unique experience. But individuals have no basis for believing or claiming, on the basis of their body's unique reactions and responses, that some risk-reducing practice or product works for them in a different way than for someone else (say, believing that he or she will have cancer prevented by Vitamin C, when aggregate data show otherwise). When it comes to risk, what we know is usually only in aggregate.

Similarly, many of us might be sympathetic to someone with terminal cancer choosing a treatment that in clinical trials showed no net benefit, or even harm. In such trials, the results might show that some individuals are helped but more are hurt. The desperate patient may have only one roll of the dice, have little concern with losing, and be willing to gamble, hoping for some remote chance of winning. But it makes little sense to allow slippage from this case to the situation of someone choosing a risk intervention for which there are reliable data showing no effect or harm. That patient is not desperate. It makes little sense to take up an ineffective or harmful practice. But sociohistorical processes have made some risks so embodied, experienced, and prevalent (the oft quoted 1:6 lifetime prevalence of prostate cancer among men or 1:8 breast cancer prevalence among women) that an individual might feel desperate enough to decide to take some screening test, despite data showing lack of efficacy, using a "logic" appropriate for people with advanced disease.[28] When it comes to decision making for many preventive practices and products, we need more surveillance of the border between disease and risk.

The cost/quality crisis in American biomedicine is typically characterized as spending more than other countries on health services without any apparent gains in objective health. Many preventive or anticipatory interventions are ineffective or only marginally effective, but costly.[29] Our policy response has largely been to encourage more and better scientific evidence and assessment, fewer perverse financial incentives, and greater consumer empowerment. Although each of these policies is important, we may also need a response that is more proactive and systemic.

Nearly a half century ago, Thomas McKeown conducted a series of influential historical studies of the epidemiological transition in which he argued that the important determinants of the decline of mortality in England and Wales had little to do with specific clinical or public health practices. Instead, the decline's origins were in nonspecific socioeconomic improvements, and largely mediated by improved nutrition. McKeown's work is sometimes misunderstood as a diatribe against all forms of medical care and focused disease prevention. It is as if his most read work, *The Role of Medicine*, should have been titled *No Role for Medicine* and as if the book's concluding chapters were not concerned with carefully distinguishing his point of view from different strains of antimedical criticism. Instead, McKeown argued that Medicine, as an institution, should shift some resources from the cure and management of acute phases of illness to the care of the symptomatically and often chronically ill.[30] He also called for more evidence-based evaluation of preventative and curative interventions, not their wholesale abandonment.

The implications McKeown drew from his analysis of the origins of the great mortality gains of the preceding century remain a relevant and valid response to the growth of health risks and risk interventions in the years since his work reached wide audiences. Medicine as an institution needs to deploy some of the extensive resources focused on risk interventions towards the care of the symptomatically and chronically ill. Moreover, there needs to be intense scientific scrutiny of risk interventions prior to the establishment of a stable risk system, when their social efficacy and other perceptions and routines can make them resistant to scientific challenge. As McKeown observed, "Once a procedure has come into general use it may be difficult, perhaps impossible to withdraw it after facilities have been provided, staff trained, and public expectations roused. However, there is a point in time when a new measure is sufficiently promising to justify its introduction on a limited scale, and when it is not yet so widely used that there are ethical and other objections to investigation of its effectiveness. If this opportunity is missed, it cannot easily be recreated, and it is for this reason that it is now difficult or impossible to assess the value of many procedures and services which have never been validated."[31]

Moreover, our current approaches to health risks may not only take up too many limited resources but sometimes permit unwarranted intrusions into the peace of mind and autonomy of individuals. The individual surveyed for risk and caught up in a web of decisions and practices about screening, behavior change, and preventive interventions often interacts with the medical system in a more uniform and less idiosyncratic way than someone with symptoms and/or active disease. The risk experience can be so uniform, quantifiable, and visible that people may be more vulnerable to unwanted surveillance and manipulation by third-party, biomedical, and government entities.

For these reasons and others, it is important to recognize the centrality of risk ideas and interventions to everyday clinical practice and consumer/patient behavior in both disease prevention and chronic disease management. Understanding and recovering the history of how such a comprehensive *risk system* developed and is sustained is a first step towards wiser and more appropriate individual and collective responses.

Acknowledgments

Risky Medicine has had a long gestation. Versions of some of the chapters were previously published. I would like to thank the following journals and publishers to reprint material (with minor changes). Chapters 2 and 5 first appeared in the *Milbank Quarterly* as "The converged experience of risk and disease," 2009, 87 (2): 417–42, and "The rise and fall of the Lyme disease vaccines: A cautionary tale for risk interventions in American medicine and public health," 2012, 90 (2): 250–77. Chapter 4 appeared as "The Framingham Heart Study and the emergence of the risk factor approach to coronary heart disease: 1947–1970," *Revue d'histoire des sciences*, 2011, 64 (2): 263–95. Chapter 6 appeared as "Gardasil: A vaccine against cancer and a drug to reduce risk," in *Three Shots at Prevention: The HPV Vaccine and the Politics of Medicine's Simple Solutions* (Baltimore: Johns Hopkins University Press, 2010), 21–38, edited by Keith Wailoo, Julie Livingston, Steven Epstein, and Robert Aronowitz. Chapter 9 appeared as "Situating risks: An opportunity for disease prevention policy," in *American Health Care History and Policy: Putting the Past Back In* (New Brunswick: Rutgers University Press, 2006), 153–65, edited by Rosemary A. Stevens, Charles E. Rosenberg, and Lawton R. Burns.

The research for this book was supported by an Investigator Award in Health Policy from the Robert Wood Johnson Foundation, a research and training grant from the Robert Wood Johnson Foundation Health & Society Scholars program at the University of Pennsylvania, and grant 1G13 LM009587-01A1 from the National Library of Medicine, NIH, and DHHS. In addition, I received financial assistance for help for final book preparation from a Research Opportunity Grant from the School of Arts and Sciences at the University of Pennsylvania. Parts of this book were drafted when I was a Visiting Scholar at the Russell Sage Foundation.

The chapters on the Framingham study and the Lyme disease vaccines could not have been written without the help of historical informants. I had extensive interviews with long-time Framingham directors Thomas R. Dawber and William Kannel, and correspondence with leading cardiovascular researcher Ancel Keys, before each of them died. Paul Offit, Stanley Plotkin, Loren Cooper, and Len Sigal offered crucial perspectives on the Lyme disease vaccine story. I would also like to thank archivists at the Countway Library (Harvard Medical School) and the National Archives who helped me find important documents, and the unnamed people who researched my Freedom of Information Act request at the National Institutes of Health.

I presented the core content and arguments of the book to different audiences in Europe and the U.S. Thank you to: Economic and Social Research Council, University of East Anglia; Social Science and Humanities Perspectives workshop, University of British Columbia; Centre de Recherche Médecine, Sciences, Santé, Santé mentale et Société (CERMES3), Paris; Science Studies colloquium, University of Oslo; the Institute of Medicine, Washington, D.C.; Max Planck Institute for Human Development, Berlin; Medical Anthropology and Human Ecology, Humboldt University, Berlin; History of Science department, Harvard; Wellcome Institute for the History and Understanding of Medicine, London; Centre for the History of Science, Medicine, and Technology at the University of Manchester; Wissenschaftszentrum Berlin fur Sozialforschung; and the Colloquium in Medical Humanities at Johns Hopkins University.

I have had research assistance from Deanna Day, Melissa Kulynych, and Molly Weisberg, and editorial advice from Kennie Lyman.

Many friends and colleagues read earlier versions of book chapters or commented on talks in which these ideas were presented. I particularly would like to thank David Barnes, Stefan Beck, Kirsten Bell, Steve Epstein, Jean-Paul Gaudillière, Élodie Giroux, Jeremy Greene, Nicolas Henckes, Annemarie Jutel, Anne Kveim-Le, Matt Liang, Susan Lindee, Beth Linker, Julie Livingston, Ilana Löwy, Projit Mukharji, Dietrich Niethammer, Jörg Niewöhner, Ohad Parnes, (the late) John

Pickstone, Svetlana Ristovski-Slijepcevic, Nick Rose, Jason Schnittker, Judy Segal, Rosemary Stevens, Andrea Stockl, Carsten Timmermans, Elizabeth Toon, Keith Wailoo, George Weiss, and Simon Wessely.

There are simply too many Robert Wood Johnson Foundation Health & Society Scholars and History and Sociology of Science graduate students at Penn to thank individually, but discussions with them over the years sharpened my arguments and made me feel there was a diverse audience for my ideas about health risks. Jason Schwartz read and commented on parts of the book focused on vaccine policies. Erica Dwyer and Luke Messac read and commented on recent draft chapters. I learned many things from working with Sejal Patel. Her own work on the Framingham and Roseto studies and the history of NIH practices influenced this book and are important complements to chapter 4.

A few close friends and colleagues have been there for the entire chronic preoccupation with risk, read drafts of different chapters, and have given me sustained and wise advice. Special thanks to David Asch, Allan Brandt, Steve Feierman, Knud Lambrecht, and Charles Rosenberg. All of my colleagues at Penn's History and Sociology of Science department have been supportive and helpful at different points in this project.

Daniel Aronowitz and Sara Aronowitz put up with my obsession with health risks over meals and family vacations. Jane Mathisen read drafts of many of these chapters, gave me thoughtful and helpful reactions as a clinician and sometimes patient/consumer, and has supported me in countless ways.

Notes

Chapter 1

1 Tara Parker-Pope, "Scientists seek to rein in diagnoses of cancer," *New York Times*, July 30, 2013, p. 1; L. J. Esserman, I. M. Thompson, and B. Reid, "Overdiagnosis and overtreatment in cancer: An opportunity for improvement," *Journal of the American Medical Association*, 2013, 310 (8): 797–98.

2 Over the past decades, anthropologists and others have done detailed ethnographic study of the experience of illness. This work has been highly influential, leading to changes in medical education and practice that encouraged clinicians to understand the cultural shaping and idiosyncratic aspects of patient's symptoms and health-related behavior. A leading practitioner and theorist, physician-anthropologist Arthur Kleinman (see, for example, his seminal *The Illness Narratives: Suffering, Healing, and the Human Condition* [New York: Basic Books, 1988]), recently offered some critical reflections on the way the "illness experience" literature has (unwittingly) contributed to simplistic deployment of "cultural competency" skills in medical education and practice, treating individual dimensions of illness as one more concrete element of everyday diagnosis and treatment, and using "fetishized illness narratives per se as symbols and stories" divorced from the economic and structural conditions that shaped them. A. Kleinman, "From illness as culture to caregiving as moral experience," *New England Journal of Medicine*, 2013, 368 (15): 1376–77).

3 J. Greene, *Prescribing by Numbers: Drugs and the Definition of Disease* (Baltimore: Johns Hopkins University Press, 2006), and S. Jasanoff, *States of Knowledge: The Co-production of Science and the Social Order* (New York: Routledge, 2006).

4 In this regard, *Risky Medicine* has some overlap with Jeremy Greene's *Prescribing by Numbers* and Joseph Dumit's *Drugs for Life: How Pharmaceutical Companies Define Our Health* (Durham, NC: Duke University Press, 2012). Some sociologists have argued that the medicalization concept has lost a good deal of its relevance and utility, e.g., J. E. Davis, "How medicalization lost its way," *Society*, 2006, 43 (6): 51–56. They note that medicalization has strayed far from its original meaning and context: the labeling of deviance as disease in order to expand medical authority. In contrast, the term *medicalization* has come to denote actions by many nonphysician actors (patients, disease advocates,

bureaucrats, drug companies, etc.) that result, through myriad processes, in the expansion of medical entities and the numbers of individuals recruited into them. While I understand the importance of recovering some conceptual clarity and political bite, social science scholarship and health policy would be poorly served if we tried to set back the clock and narrow the term's scope. It is not simply that the sociologists' *concept* has expanded in the intervening years. Rather, there has been a transformation in how ill health has been produced, labeled, managed, and ultimately experienced.

5 This and related ideas that follow in the next few pages are largely excerpted from R. Aronowitz, "Framing disease: an underappreciated mechanism for the social patterning of health," *Social Science & Medicine*, 2008, 67 (1): 1–9.

6 See also N. Tomes, "Merchants of health: medicine and consumer culture in the United States, 1900–1940," *Journal of American History*, 2001, 88 (2): 519–47, and A. Brandt, *The Cigarette Century: The Rise, Fall, and Deadly Persistence of the Product That Defined America* (New York: Basic Books, 2007).

7 N. Schull, "Digital gambling: the coincidence of desire and design," *Annals of the American Academy of Political and Social Science*, 2005, 597 (1): 65–81. See also Schull's *Addiction by Design: Machine Gambling in Las Vegas* (Princeton: Princeton University Press, 2012).

8 M. Richtel, "Wasting time is new divide in digital era," *New York Times*, May 30, 2012, A1.

9 I. Hacking, "The looping effects of human kinds," in D. Sperber, D. Premack, and A. J. Premack, eds., *Causal Cognition: A Multi-disciplinary Approach* (Oxford: Clarendon Press, 1995), 351–82.

10 C. E. Rosenberg, "Pathologies of progress: the idea of civilization as risk," *Bulletin of the History of Medicine*, Winter 1998, 72 (4): 714–30.

11 W. Labov, "The social stratification of (r) in New York City department stores," in *Sociolinguistic Patterns* (Philadelphia: University of Pennsylvania Press, 1972), 43–54.

12 P. Bourdieu, *Distinction: A Social Critique of the Judgement of Taste*, trans. R. Nice (Cambridge: Harvard University Press, 1987).

13 S. A. Grier and S. Kumanyika, "Targeted marketing and public health," *Annual Review of Public Health*, 2010, 31: 349–69.

14 R. Aronowitz, *Making Sense of Illness: Science, Society, and Disease* (Cambridge, U.K.: Cambridge University Press, 1998); G. Rose, "Sick individuals and sick populations," *International Journal of Epidemiology*, 1985, 14 (1): 32–38. Individual risk assessment may also be an inefficient and unscientific way to promote change relevant for an entire population. Public television recently aired a documentary on personalized genomics. The program had a segment with Francis Collins, a physician-scientist who happens to be the current NIH director. Collins had his genome sequenced and was told that he had a modestly increased relative risk for type 2 diabetes. The importance of screening was indicated by Collins' use of this genetic variation as motivation to lose 27 lbs. Is this the appropriate message? If Collins believes averting type 2 diabetes and cardiovascular disease (the most common serious consequence of diabetes) is important and that weight loss is a reasonable means, why does he need the evidence of increased genetic risk to motivate him? Most everyone knows that weight gain is a risk factor for type 2 diabetes. Type 2 diabetes is becoming a mass disease and cardiovascular disease is already one, affecting some half of the male population. Weight loss is a good practice for all kinds of reasons, and not just for people at high risk of heart disease. Transcript of "Crack Your Genetic Code," originally broadcast on PBS March 28, 2012, available at http://

www.pbs.org/wgbh/nova/body/cracking-your-genetic-code.html, accessed
July 2014.

15 M. Foucault, *The Birth of Biopolitics: Lectures at the Collège de France 1978–1979,*
    trans. G. Burchell (Basingstoke: Palgrave Macmillan, 2008); J. Scott, *Seeing Like
    a State: How Certain Schemes to Improve the Human Condition Have Failed* (New
    Haven: Yale University Press, 2008); D. Armstrong, "The rise of surveillance
    medicine," *Sociology of Health and Illness,* 1995, 17 (3): 393–404.

Chapter 2

1 J. Greene, *Prescribing by Numbers: Drugs and the Definition of Disease* (Baltimore:
   Johns Hopkins University Press, 2006).

2 D. Armstrong, "The rise of surveillance medicine," *Sociology of Health and Illness,* 1995, 17 (3): 393–404.

3 A. Barsky, *Worried Sick: Our Troubled Quest for Wellness* (Boston: Little, Brown,
   1998).

4 See, for example, U. Beck, *Risk Society: Towards a New Modernity* (London:
   Sage, 1992), and A. Giddens, *The Consequences of Modernity* (Stanford: Stanford
   University Press, 1990).

5 M. Klawiter, "Risk, prevention, and the breast cancer continuum: the NCI, the
   FDA, health activism, and the pharmaceutical industry," *History and Technology,*
   2002, 18: 309–53.

6 See C. Feudtner, "Disease in motion: diabetes history and the new paradigm
   of transmuted disease," *Perspectives in Biology and Medicine* 1996, 39 (Winter):
   158–70. My focus on the risky nature of chronic disease is related to Feudtner's
   concept of a *transmuted* chronic disease. Feudtner stressed the shift from the
   experience of a stable, external, and specific "natural history" to something
   more dynamic, individual, and negotiated. For the subset of patients with a
   chronic disease diagnosis for whom an "early" diagnosis and medical intervention have rendered them at least temporarily asymptomatic, there has been a
   paradoxical return to a stable, although more anticipated than experienced,
   natural history.

7 R. Aronowitz, *Unnatural History: Breast Cancer and American Society* (Cambridge, U.K.: Cambridge University Press, 2007).

8 National Digestive Diseases Information Clearing House. 2008. Information
   Sheet. Available at http://digestive.niddk.nih.gov/ddiseases/pubs/chronichepc
   /index.htm (accessed May 2008).

9 Very recently, quicker acting, safer, and highly effective oral treatments
   against hepatitis C have been marketed. These improvements promise to
   shift rather than eliminate individual or societal dilemmas. At an estimated
   charge of $84,000 for a twelve-week course of pills, insurers, clinicians, and
   patients face difficult decisions about who will pay and who will be denied
   access.

10 C. Novas and N. Rose, "Genetic risk and the birth of the somatic individual,"
    Economy and Society, 2000, 29: 485–513.

11 P. D. Kramer, *Listening to Prozac* (New York: Penguin, 1993).

12 L. Ries, M. P. Eisner, C. L. Kosary, B. F. Hankey, B. A. Miller, L. Clegg, A. Mari-
    otto, E. J. Feuer, and B. K. Edwards, eds, *SEER Cancer Statistics Review, 1975–
    2002* (Bethesda, Md.: National Cancer Institute, 2005). Available at http://
    seer.cancer.gov/csr/1975_2002/, based on November 2004 SEER data sub-
    mission, posted to the SEER website 2005 (accessed July 25, 2008).

13 E. Rosenthal, "Drugs can prevent diabetes in many at high risk, study suggests," *New York Times*, September 17, 2006, A1.

14 R. Aronowitz, "Do not delay: breast cancer and time, 1900–1970," *Milbank Quarterly* 2001, 79 (3): 355–86.

15 L. Schwartz, S. Woloshin, F. J. Fowler, and H. G. Welch, "Enthusiasm for cancer screening in the United States," *Journal of American Medical Association*, 2004, 291 (1): 71–78.

16 Adapted from E. Goffman, *Asylums: Essays on the Social Situation of Mental Patients and Other Inmates* (Garden City, N.Y.: Doubleday, 1961).

17 Surveillance, Epidemiology, and End Results (SEER), 2008, available at http://dccps.nci.nih.gov/ocs/prevalence/prevalence.html (accessed March 2008). For an interesting discussion of what he characterizes as a "remission society," see A. W. Frank, *The Wounded Storyteller: Body, Illness, and Ethics* (Chicago: University of Chicago Press, 1995).

18 http://www.survivorshipguidelines.org/pdf/ltfuguidelines.pdf; accessed December 29, 2014.

19 F. E. Johnson, Y. Maehara, G. P. Browman, J. A. Margenthaler, R. A. Audisio, J. F. Thompson, D. Y. Johnson, C. C. Earle, and K. Virgo, *Patient Surveillance after Cancer Treatment* (New York: Springer, 2013).

20 A. Pollack, "FDA reviews arthritis drugs for links to cancer," *New York Times*, June 5, 2008, C2.

21 See C. E. Rosenberg, "The tyranny of diagnosis: specific entities and individual experience," *Milbank Quarterly*, 2002, 80 (2): 237–60; C. E. Rosenberg, "What is disease? In memory of Oswei Temkin," *Bulletin of the History of Medicine*, 2003, 77: 491–505; and C. E. Rosenberg, "Managed fear," *Lancet*, 2009, 373: 802–3.

22 Aronowitz, *Unnatural History*.

23 T. M. Tuttle, E. B. Habermann, E. H. Grund, T. J. Morris, and B. A. Virnig, "Increasing use of contralateral prophylactic mastectomy for breast cancer patients: a trend toward more aggressive surgical treatment," *Journal of Clinical Oncology*, 2007, 25 (33): 5203–9.

24 I have been unable to date to find good (i.e., population-based) data on temporal trends in prophylactic bilateral mastectomy rates among women without breast cancer. One study used a database of women who had mutations for BRCA1 and BRCA2 and reported that American women had the highest rates of prophylactic surgery (36.3 percent) among the nine industrialized countries they compared. K. A. Metcalfe, D. Birenbaum-Carmeli, J. Lubinski, J. Gronwald, H. Lynch, P. Moller, P. Ghadirian, W. D. Foulkes, J. Klijn, E. Friedman, C. Kim-Sing, P. Ainsworth, B. Rosen, S. Domchek, T. Wagner, N. Tung, S. Manoukian, F. Couch, P. Sun, S. A. Narod, and the Hereditary Breast Cancer Clinical Study Group, "International Variation in Rates of Uptake of Preventive Options in BRCA1 and BRCA2 Mutation Carriers," *International Journal of Cancer*, 2008, 122 (9): 2017–22.

25 In stage 1 breast cancer, the cancer has not spread beyond the breast and is no more than 2 cm wide; in stage 2, the cancer is between 2 and 5 cm wide; and in stage 3, the cancer is larger than 5 cm and has spread to the lymph nodes or local tissues.

26 A. Pollack, "Study links rise in mastectomies to M.R.I. detection," *New York Times*, May 16, 2008, A16.

27 Type 1 and type 2 diabetes are distinct diseases with different pathological bases, and it is likely that this actress was misdiagnosed if she were truly able to wean herself off insulin by dietary or other behavioral change. Whether sci-

entifically accurate or not, however, the expansion of diabetes continuum is a very real phenomenon.

Chapter 3

1 C. Rosenberg, "The therapeutic revolution: medicine, meaning and social change in nineteenth-century America," *Perspectives in Biology and Medicine*, 1977, 20 (4): 485–506. I link performativity and ritual to underscore that therapeutics does social and psychological work, i.e., real, not solely or mostly, symbolic action. Rosenberg explained that the term "exhibition" captured the way the administration and receipt of drugs reinforced the social ties between traditional healer and patient, in a period in which therapy occurred in the home and whose details—often mixtures of herbs and chemicals tailored for the individual patient—were ideally shaped by a long-term relationship between these actors. Parenthetically, a great deal of modern anthropological and other scholarship on ritual has similarly emphasized—on both substantive and theoretical grounds—the actual social and psychological work done by specific rituals over symbolic and functionalist explanations. See W. Sax, J. Quack, and J. Weinhold, eds., *The Problem of Ritual Efficacy* (New York: Oxford University Press, 2010). A similar line of criticism could be advanced about the narrow confines within which placebo efficacy is evaluated. Typically placebos are understood to work either by somatic mechanisms (usually understood in terms of mind-body connectivity by numerous and constantly changing neurological and hormonal mediators) or suggestion and other purely psychological mechanisms. But it may be that placebos have more social and psychological efficacy, e.g., they convince people in the control arm of an antidepressant trial that their doctors care about them, which brightens their mood, which is then observed and registered as a placebo effect.

2 In recent years, demographers and others have tried to characterize and quantify this net vector with concepts such as allostatic load, a composite score constituted by a hodgepodge of historical, laboratory, and clinical variables thought to be associated with the body's wear and tear.

3 R. Aronowitz, *Unnatural History: Breast Cancer and American Society* (Cambridge, U.K.: Cambridge University Press, 2007).

4 In June 2009, the Institute of Medicine issued a policy brief on their Comparative Effectiveness initiative, which estimated that there is inadequate evidence for half of all current medical interventions. See http://www.iom.edu/~/media/Files/Report%20Files/2009/ComparativeEffectivenessResearchPriorities/CER%20report%20brief%2008-13-09.ashx, accessed on June 8, 2012.

5 The situation is often framed in a similar way to how doctors understand patient deviations from their orders as *noncompliance*. In this noncompliance framework, the focus is on what patients do not do. A more insightful approach is to ask what patients *are* doing. Understood this way, one can see more clearly the determinants of individual behavior, as Anne Fadiman did in her study of a Hmong immigrant family's struggle to do the best thing with their daughter's severe and medically recalcitrant epilepsy. See A. Fadiman, *The Spirit Catches You and You Fall Down* (New York: Farrar, Straus and Giroux, 1998).

6 Most relevant are the reviews by S. R. Whyte, S. van der Geest, and A. Hardon, *Social Lives of Medicines* (Cambridge: Cambridge University Press, 2002), and by N. Vuckovic and M. Nichter, "Changing patterns of pharmaceutical practice in the United States," *Social Science & Medicine*, 1997, 44: 1285–1302.

7   Whyte, van der Geest, and Hardon, *Social Lives of Medicines*, also includes drug manufacturers within its ethnographic gaze but notes that it is very difficult to directly observe them. The authors rightly stress that pharmaceutical companies not only make drugs, but also manufacture their meaning and drum up demand for them.

8   See H. M. Marks, *The Progress of Experiment: Science and Therapeutic Reform in the United States, 1900–1990* (Cambridge, U.K.: Cambridge University Press, 1997), and S. Reverby, "Stealing the golden eggs: Ernest Amory Codman and the science and management of medicine," *Bulletin of the History of Medicine*, 55 (Summer 1981): 156–71.

9   Insufficient scholarly attention has been directed to historical changes in how medical efficacy is understood and constructed. S. Shapin, "Possessed by the Idols" (book review), *London Review of Books*, 2006, 28 (23): 31–33, pointed out that efficacy itself has not been sufficiently historicized. "Historians should be interested in what counts as working, and how that's changed." See also Rosenberg, "Therapeutic revolution."

10 Aronowitz, *Unnatural History*.

11 See my *Unnatural History* and I. Löwy, *Prevention Strikes: Women, Cancer, and Prophylactic Surgery* (Baltimore: Johns Hopkins University Press, 2010), for more elaboration of embodied risk.

12 Transient HPV infection, often without signs or symptoms, occurs in most everyone in the first years of active sexual life.

13 For most women, HPV infection is asymptomatic. Women know they have HPV infection because of an abnormal Pap or HPV screening test.

14 http://www.gardasil.com/gardasil-information/i-chose/, accessed March 29, 2012.

15 A similar logic can hold for situations in which the issue is not avoiding a risk state but the uncertainty and incompleteness of treatments that promise control rather than elimination of disease. Some people shift from medical treatment of underlying coronary artery disease (beta blockers, treatment of high cholesterol and hypertension, antianginal medications) to coronary bypass surgery because surgery promises a more definitive cure. They hope to avoid the limbo state that seemingly halfway measures create. Another intervention that promises definitive rather than halfway results is corrective Lasik surgery.

16 S. B. Thacker, D. Stroup, and C. Man-huei, "Continuous electronic heart rate monitoring for fetal assessment during labor," *Cochrane Database of Systematic Reviews*, 2006; http://onlinelibrary.wiley.com/doi/10.1002/14651858.CD 000063.pub2/abstract, accessed February 13, 2013.

17 *Continuous* monitoring is also appealing because it appears to be more *complete*, i.e., more thorough and with reduced probability of missing an actionable sign. In this way, this technology's social and psychological efficacy is similar to other risk interventions such as screening colonoscopy, which provides a complete survey of the colon. This procedure is generally preferred over the more (anatomically) limited flexible sigmoidoscopy, which had once been promoted as a cost-effective screening with very limited success. Similar to my argument about continuous monitoring of fetal heart sounds, the work of reassurance is more easily accomplished by a screening technology that surveys the entire area of potential risk over one that gives only a partial look.

18 In 2012 the results of a well-done clinical trial were released online that provided crucial medical evidence for the efficacy of taking Tamoxifen for an additional five years for some women. See C. Davies, H. Pan, J. Godwin, R. Gray, R. Arriagada, et al., "Long-term effects of continuing adjuvant tamoxifen

to 10 years versus stopping at 5 years after diagnosis of oestrogen receptor-positive breast cancer: ATLAS, a randomised trial," *Lancet*, 2013, 381 (9869): 805–16. The demand for longer courses of treatment existed—and exists—independently of the scientific evidence for this practice.

19 One study argued that while statistically significant, the amount of average improvement—over a presumed worse decline—associated with putatively effective Alzheimer interventions was clinically insignificant. The degree of average change on standardized measures would not be reliably noticed by a clinician. R. E. Becker and S. Markwell, "Problems arising from the generalizing of treatment efficacy from clinical trials in Alzheimer's disease," *Clinical Drug Investigation*, 2000, 19: 33–41. Clinicians and drug companies do not conspire to obscure this minimal benefit. Many individuals or their families probably sign on for a trial of Aricept hoping to "win the lottery." Instead of expecting the average clinically insignificant benefit, they hope for the more remote chance of a significant benefit.

20 I am focusing on sociostructural aspects of persuasion rather than the individual psychological dimension to risk decisions. An entire field of behavioral economics has developed around decision making under uncertainty that focuses on this individual dimension. See D. Kahneman, P. Slovic, and A. Tversky, eds., *Judgment under Uncertainty: Heuristics and Biases* (New York: Cambridge University Press, 1982).

21 I am making a distinction between persuasion by evidence qua evidence and persuasion by stylized performances of evidence production and meaningfulness. Both have been operative in persuading researchers, clinicians, patients, and consumers that some risk interventions work. But in many ways the distinction is artificial, at least historically. The creation and interpretation of scientific evidence has long had performative qualities. Steven Shapin and Simon Schaffer, in their groundbreaking *Leviathan and the Air-Pump: Hobbes, Boyle, and the Experimental Life* (Princeton: Princeton University Press, 1985), convincingly trace the origins of modern experimental science from the direct and public witnessing of Boyle's air pump by esteemed, well-respected members of an elite group of natural philosophers who had high mutual trust to the more virtual witnessing through scientific publications and the creation of more formal and geographically spread out communities of experts. Persuasion by evidence necessarily involves trust, assessment of credibility, and stylized means of exhibiting data. Nevertheless, there remains a fundamental difference between the pitches made in, say, direct-to-consumer advertising (DTCA) and the persuasion that follows from expert reviews of high-quality scientific evidence. DTCA pitches have a lot more in common with toothpaste advertisements than the virtual witnessing that is constitutive of modern medical journals and scientific reports.

22 In the era before DTCA, two physician friends sent inquiries to drug companies who sponsored print advertisements for their medicines in medical journals that contained claims of efficacy and safety and a note promising that "additional references were available on request." Very few of the companies responded to the request for additional information. A reasonable interpretation of this low response rate is that the companies had no expectation that anyone would actually take them up on their offer to provide further references (David Asch, personal communication, June 2012).

23 N. Tomes, "The great American medicine show revisited," *Bulletin of the History of Medicine*, 2005, 79: 627–63.

24 See the extensive online collection of early twentieth-century Listerine print

advertisements organized by Duke University, e.g., http://library.duke.edu
/digitalcollections/mma_MM0633/`, accessed May 2012. In this and other
1930s advertisements, quantitative claims as if from laboratory and epidemiological study were made about Listerine's bacteria-killing qualities. "Laboratory tests show that it kills even such stubborn disease-producing organisms
as the Staphylococcus Auereus (pus) and Bacillus Typhosus (typhoid) in counts
ranging to 100,000,000 in 15 seconds. We could not make this statement
unless we were prepared to prove it to the entire satisfaction of the medical
profession and the U.S. Government." Medical credibility—attested to by support of the medical community—was crucial to establishing the product's efficacy. Another 1930 advertisement proclaimed, "A billion dollars couldn't buy
this endorsement—The mighty Lancet approves Listerine." http://library.duke
.edu/digitalcollections/mma_MM0625/, accessed May 2012. Other Listerine
advertisements deployed clinical trial results similar to the Crest commercials discussed here, e.g., "Let the tests speak for themselves: Of 102 persons
observed for a period of seventy-five days, one-third, known as 'controls,' did
not gargle with Listerine at all; one-third gargled twice a day; the other third
five times a day, the full strength solution. Now, note these amazing results:
those who did not gargle, contracted twice as many colds as those who gargled
Listerine twice a day. The colds were four times as severe and lasted three times
as long." "Controlled test on 102 people shows 1/2 As Many Colds For Listerine
Users," available at http://library.duke.edu/digitalcollections/mma_MM0649/,
undated, accessed May 2012.

25 These Crest commercials accompanied NBC's presentation of *What Makes
Sammy Run?* in 1959, shown in two parts on its *Sunday Showcase* series. I
obtained a copy of the original video that included these commercials from the
producers of the 2009 DVD release of the original program (which omits these
commercials); thanks to Ed Tepper at Mongo Media, New York.

26 A. Brandt, *The Cigarette Century: The Rise, Fall, and Deadly Persistence of the Product That Defined America* (New York: Basic Books, 2007).

27 For a seminal sociological formulation of reflexivity, see R. K. Merton, "The
self-fulfilling prophecy," *Antioch Review*, 1948, 8: 193–210. I find the Wikipedia
entry for "reflexivity" clear and helpful as well: "Reflexivity is considered to
occur when the observations or actions of observers in the social system affect
the very situations they are observing, or theory being formulated is disseminated to and affects the behaviour of the individuals or systems the theory is
meant to be objectively modelling. Thus for example an anthropologist living
in an isolated village may affect the village and the behaviour of its citizens that
he or she is studying. The observations are not independent of the participation of the observer." http://en.wikipedia.org/wiki/Reflexivity_(social_theory),
accessed July 2014.

28 See also Hacking on the similar phenomenon he labels *looping* effects, e.g.,
I. Hacking, "The looping effects of human kinds," in D. Sperber and A. Premark,
eds., *Causal Cognition: A Multi-disciplinary Approach* (Oxford: Clarendon Press,
1995), 351–94.

29 L. Fleck, *Genesis and Development of a Scientific Fact*, translated by F. Bradley
and T. J. Trenn (Chicago: University of Chicago Press, 1979), xxviii.

30 George Soros, "The crisis and what to do about it," *New York Review of Books*,
December 4, 2008, 55 (19): 63–65; R. Aronowitz, "Do not delay: breast cancer
and time, 1900–1970," *Milbank Quarterly*, 2001, 79: 355–86.

31 Consumers of risk-reducing pills sometimes seek additional witnessed evidence that a drug or preventive practice has had some effect on the body. For

example, patients may find something positive in a rash or fever after vaccination, understanding this change as evidence that a vaccine has been "taken"
by the body. Although typically without clear clinical indications, physicians
sometimes order serum antibody tests to determine whether a hepatitis B
immunization has "taken."

32 There is a much longer history of what might be called the rise of "medium
endpoints," which is coterminous with modern invasive therapeutics. In breast
cancer, for example, William Halsted promoted his radical cancer surgery
largely on the basis of evidence that it resulted in better local control of cancer.
Local control was an intermediate endpoint, important in many ways, but not
equivalent to cure or longer life, neither of which were produced by radical surgery. See Aronowitz, *Unnatural History*. To take an example from modern cancer therapeutics, clinicians often speak of "complete remissions" from chemotherapy, by which they mean not cure or prolonged life, but evidence that the
existing signs of cancer have disappeared. The kind of efficacy promoted by
Halsted for his complete operations and modern use of "complete remissions"
often lead to difficult ambiguity between patient and doctor, where the words
suggest more important and significant types of efficacy than they actually
denote. Both types of efficacy claims also serve as a promissory note within the
progress of therapeutics, suggesting they are a kind of down payment on future
"real cures."

33 G. Kolata, "Experts reshape treatment guide for cholesterol," *New York Times*,
November 12, 2013, A1.

Chapter 4

1 R. Knox, "Private gifts revive Framingham heart study," *Boston Globe*, March 7,
1971, 63.

2 For example, J. T. Doyle, A. S. Heslin, H. E. Hilleboe, P. F. Formel, and R. F.
Korns, "A prospective study of degenerative cardiovascular disease in Albany:
Report of three years' experience—I. Ischemic heart disease," *American Journal
of Public Health*, 1957, 47 (4, supplement): 25–32. Unlike the epidemiological
study in Albany, Framingham enrolled both women and men.

3 For some of the most recent scholarship see H. M. Marks, *The Progress of Experiment: Science and Therapeutic Reform in the United States, 1900–1990* (Cambridge,
U.K.: Cambridge University Press, 1997); S. Patel, "The eclipse of the community study: The Roseto study in historical context," Ph.D. dissertation, University of Pennsylvania, retrieved April 15, 2010, from Dissertations & Theses: Full
Text (Publication No. AAT 3271797). See also E. Giroux, "Origines de l'étude
prospective de cohorte: Épidémiologie cardio-vasculaire américaine et étude
de Framingham," *Revue d'histoire des sciences*, 2011, 64 (2): 297–318 (and other
articles in that special issue, which was devoted to the history of risk factors).

4 M. Susser, "Epidemiology in the United States after World War II: The Evolution of Technique," *Epidemiology, Health & Society: Selected Papers of Mervyn
Susser* (New York: Oxford University Press, 1987), 22–49, 32. Susser argued
that twentieth-century epidemiological methods "flowed from a succession of
designs tried in the field—cross-sectional field survey, cohort, retrospective
case-control, quasi-experimental, and experimental—in an intriguing dialectic
evolution" (p. 27).

5 B. Bullough and G. Rosen, *Preventive Medicine in the United States, 1900–1990*
(Canton, MA: Science History Publications, 1992), 26.

6   For an overview of this early TB project, see George W Comstock's "Commentary: The first Framingham Study—a pioneer in community-based participatory research (reprint)," *International Journal of Epidemiology* (2005) 34: 1188–90.

7   To contrast the resources set aside for heart disease control as opposed to clinical and laboratory research, in 1948 Congress allocated $250,000 for state control programs at the same time $1 million was set aside for heart disease research fellowships and $25 million for construction of heart disease research facilities (minutes of the National Advisory Heart Council [NAHC] meeting held on September 8, 1948, record group 443, stack area 3w2b, row 46, Records of the National Institutes of Health, National Archives, Washington, D.C.). Individual state grants for cardiac control were all under $33,000 (ibid., minutes of NAHC meeting, December 10–11, 1948).

8   In 1949, the NAHC reviewed the results of the National Health Survey and concluded that they showed the "the inadequacies of our knowledge of the heart disease problem." Framingham is offered up as a corrective not only for contributing to better statistics, but to give "some idea of the amount of cardiovascular disease which can be uncovered in a general population by a fairly comprehensive examination." Ibid, minutes of NAHC meeting, October 24–25, 1950.

9   Commission on Chronic Illness, *Prevention of Chronic Illness in the United States*, vol. 1 (Cambridge, MA: Harvard University Press, for the Commonwealth Fund, 1957), 157.

10 Both William Kannel (personal communication, May 5, 1995) and Ancel Keys (personal communication, December 15, 1991) claimed that the USPHS was inspired to start Framingham as a direct consequence of Keys' early studies. Keys was a seminal figure in many medical developments in addition to helping to establish the diet-heart disease connection, e.g., in exercise physiology and nutrition ("K-rations"). Sarah Tracy is currently completing a biography of Keys.

11 R. Aronowitz "From the patient's angina pectoris to the cardiologist's coronary heart disease," in *Making Sense of Illness: Science, Society, and Disease* (Cambridge, U.K.: Cambridge University Press, 1998), 84–110.

12 See W. R. Houston, "The spasmogenic aptitude," *Medical Clinics of North America*, 1929, 12: 1285–1302.

13 W. D. Stroud, *Diagnosis and Treatment of Cardiovascular Disease* (Philadelphia: F. A. Davis, 1950), esp. 1159–63.

14 Thomas Dawber, personal communication, January 20, 1997.

15 Copy of plan agreed to by Meadors, Getting, and Rutstein on December 10, 1947. Obtained from the files of the Office of Biometry through a "freedom of information" request to the NIH (hereafter FOI). See G. Oppenheimer, "Becoming the Framingham Study, 1947–1950," *American Journal of Public Health*, April 2005, 95 (4): 602–10, for a similar account that gives more detail and greater emphasis to the efforts of Mountin, Meadors, and, Rutstein.

16 Massachusetts Medical Society, Minutes of meeting, *New England Journal of Medicine*, 1948, 239: 130.

17 Copy of plan agreed to by Meadors, Getting, and Rutstein on December 10, 1947 (FOI). During the first year of planning, NIH investigators planned a second study in nearby Newton, Massachusetts, that would concentrate on the more practical aspects of cardiac control. In effect, this allowed Framingham to evolve into a more bona fide research study. Memorandum from Meadors to the Chief, Heart Disease Demonstration Section, at Temple University, January 8, 1948 (FOI).

18 The U.S. Public Health service had previously given support to Dr. Bert Boone
    to develop the electrokymograph at Temple University. Meadors planned to
    test the utility of this device at Framingham. Memo from Meadors to the Chief,
    Heart Disease Demonstration Section, at Temple University, January 8, 1948,
    FOI. The electrokymograph was listed as part of the clinic routine in the Heart
    Disease Epidemiologic Study, Manual of Operation, November 1, 1949, a copy
    of which was kept with the personal records of Paul Dudley White (Countway
    Historical Collection, HMS c36, box 37, folder 12). Sometime in 1949–50, this
    device seems to have been dropped from routine examinations. According to
    Dawber (personal communication, January 20, 1997), this device was an espe-
    cially poor candidate for screening because it was cumbersome and compli-
    cated.

19 These details are discussed in two early memos from Meadors to Dr. Boone
    (chief, Heart Disease Demonstration Section) dated January 8, 1948, and
    November 1, 1948, FOI. The detail about first enrolling Framingham physicians
    comes from Thomas Dawber, personal communication, January 20, 1997. See
    also Oppenheimer, "Becoming the Framingham study," for additional details
    about how the study was appealing to a group of "young Turk" community
    physicians who had moved to Framingham in the 1930s as well as details about
    different community committees who advised and supported the study.

20 Van Slyke also was involved in the now infamous Guatemalan syphilis experi-
    ments conducted by USPHS researchers. See S. Reverby, "'Normal Exposure'
    and Inoculation Syphilis: A PHS 'Tuskegee' Doctor in Guatemala, 1946–48,"
    Journal of Policy History 23 (Winter 2011): 6–28 and the Presidential Commis-
    sion for the Study of Bioethical Issues, "'Ethically Impossible' STD Research in
    Guatemala from 1946 to 1948," available online at http://bioethics.gov/sites
    /default/files/Ethically-Impossible_PCSBI.pdf, accessed August 15, 2013.

21 Memorandum from Van Slyke to Meadors, dated August 20, 1949, FOI.

22 Thomas Dawber, personal communication, January 20, 1997. See Oppen-
    heimer, "Becoming the Framingham study," for more detail on Rutstein's role
    in Framingham's reorganization.

23 Most of these details are present in a memo from Van Slyke to Meadors, dated
    August 30, 1949, FOI.

24 Memo from Meadors to Dr. Vlado Getting, dated September 19, 1949, FOI.

25 See J. McKenzie, *The basis of vital activity: being a review of five years' work at the
    St. Andrews Institute for Clinical Research* (London: Faber and Gwyer, 1926).

26 Thomas Dawber, personal communication, January 20, 1997.

27 E. O. Wheeler, P. D. White, E. W. Reed, and M. E. Cohen, "Neurocirculatory
    asthenia (anxiety neurosis, effort syndrome, neurasthenia): A twenty year
    follow-up study of one hundred and seventy-three patients," *Journal of the
    American Medical Association*, 1950: 878–89.

28 Paul D. White, "The cardiologist enlists the epidemiologist," *American Journal of
    Public Health* 47 (1957)4, Suppl.: 1–3.

29 Dawber recollected that it would have been a "bad public relations thing if they
    had excluded anybody." Personal communication, January 20, 1997.

30 While it is not at all clear that Framingham avoided the appearance of service
    either to individuals or to the community, such explicit disavowals were fre-
    quently offered to dampen the traditional suspicion of private doctors and lay
    persons in the community. Memorandum from Meadors to Van Slyke, dated
    September 19, 1949, FOI.

31 Dawber, personal communication, January 20, 1997.

32 *Heart Disease Epidemiology Study: Manual of Operation.*

33 T. R. Dawber, G. F. Meadors, and F. E. Moore, "Epidemiological approaches to

heart disease: the Framingham study," *American Journal of Public Health* 1951, 41 (3): 279–86.

34 The original Framingham manual listed twenty-seven specific hypotheses, including ones such as that "excessive and neurotic concern over manifestations of cardiac action (neurocirculatory asthenia and cardiac neurosis) affect the age of onset and rate of progression of degenerative cardiovascular disease." *Heart Disease Epidemiology Study: Manual of Operation.* These hypotheses led to forty-four categories of historical information and fifty-nine different parts to the physical examination and general impressions, in addition to objective testing such as EKGs and cholesterol determinations. In order to carry out this study on thousands of individuals and record reliable and codeable information, this initial framework required substantial revision. Framingham investigators also wrestled with the choice of endpoints. While the study purported to examine the role of different factors on the development of coronary atherosclerosis, coronary atherosclerosis could not be examined directly (excepting the few cases that came to autopsy). The end points for an epidemiological study were by necessity proxy measures. To this day, some of the inconsistencies in CHD epidemiologic studies and clinical trials have been explained by the fact that the underlying processes of interest, atherosclerosis and thrombosis, were never directly measured but rather their clinical manifestations, adding an unavoidable imprecision to results. "The difficulty of diagnosing arteriosclerotic heart disease, underestimated by some, will no doubt continue to obscure the evaluation of causal relationships." T. R. Dawber, F. E. Moore, and G. V. Mann, "Coronary heart disease in the Framingham study," *American Journal of Public Health*, 1957, 47 (4, supplement): 4–24.

35 Dawber was not moved by contemporary proponents of the "stress causes heart disease" idea or more generally by the then popular psychosomatic movement. Dawber visited Philadelphia in the 1950s to consult with Edward Weiss and O. Spurgeon English, leading figures in the psychosomatic movement. Despite the then popular slogan "tension, tension, hypertension," Dawber recalls that these luminaries were unsure if psychosomatic diseases, of which hypertension was sometimes thought paradigmatic, truly existed. Thomas Dawber, personal communication, January 20, 1997.

36 Dietary studies were later done on subsets of the Framingham study population.

37 For a clear exposition of Framingham's methodological shortcomings see T. Gordon, F. E. Moore, D. D. Shurtleff, and T. R. Dawber, "Some methodological problems in the long-term study of cardiovascular disease: observations on the Framingham study," *Journal of Chronic Disease*, 1959, 10: 186–206. The authors give an impassioned defense of the importance of community studies even if they introduce biases less evident in clinical trials and laboratory medicine.

38 Thomas Dawber, personal communication, January 20, 1997.

39 Report of the conference on epidemiology of atherosclerosis and hypertension, held at Arden House, Harriman, N.Y., January 29–February 2, 1956; American Heart Association booklet.

40 Dawber recalled (personal communication, January 20, 1997) that both he and the staff were frustrated by the lack of publications but that Van Slyke insisted that they hold off publishing any data until they could say something important about the development of CHD. Dawber felt that Van Slyke was under intense pressure to justify the length and expense of Framingham and that the publication of merely descriptive results or methodological details would feed Framingham's critics. In retrospect, Dawber believed that Van Slyke was right to hold off on publications and that the Framingham investigators were lucky that the original follow-up conclusions were later corroborated by later data.

41 Memorandum from Thomas D. Dublin, medical director, community services programs at NIH, to the director, NHI, dated March 1, 1956, FOI.

42 Memorandum from Thomas R. Dawber to James Watt, director, National Heart Institute, dated April 4, 1956, FOI.

43 Thomas Dawber, personal communication, January 20, 1997.

44 Dawber, Moore, and Mann, "Coronary heart disease in the Framingham study."

45 Dawber, Moore, and Mann, "Coronary heart disease in the Framingham study."

46 J. T. Doyle, A. S. Heslin, H. E. Hilleboe, P. F. Formel, and R. F. Korns, "A prospective study of degenerative cardiovascular disease in Albany: report of three years' experience—I. ischemic heart disease," *American Journal of Public Health*, 1957, 47 (4, supplement): 25–32; R. M. Drake, R. W. Buechley, and L. Breslow, "An epidemiological investigation of coronary heart disease in the California health survey population," *American Journal of Public Health*, 1957, 47 (4, supplement): 43–57.

47 Bibliography of Framingham Study prepared by Dr. Robert Garrison, July 28, 1994, for the NHI Office of Biometry, July 28, 1994. See the Framingham website for a more up-to-date chronology of the much greater number of more recent Framingham reports: http://www.framinghamheartstudy.org/biblio/index.html.

48 William Kannel, personal correspondence, May 1995.

49 W. B. Kannel, T. R. Dawber, A. Kagan, N. Revotskie, and J. Stokes III, "Factors of risk in the development of coronary heart disease: six-year follow-up experience—the Framingham study," *Annals of Internal Medicine* 55 (1961) 1: 33–50. William Rothstein has pointed out that related terminology was used by life insurers earlier in the century. W. Rothstein, "The development of the concept of the risk factor," paper presented to the 68th Annual Meeting of the American Association for the History of Medicine, Pittsburgh, PA, May 12, 1995. See also W. Rothstein, *Public Health and the Risk Factor: A History of an Uneven Medical Revolution* (Rochester: University of Rochester Press, 2003). Of course, there were many approximations to this term in earlier Framingham publications but my extensive reading of medical and lay publications up to this time has not shown an earlier use of the two words used as a noun compound.

50 T. R. Dawber, W. B. Kannel, and P. McNamara, "The prediction of coronary heart disease," in S. R. Moore, ed., *Transactions of the Association of Life Insurance Medical Directors of America, 72nd Annual Meeting* (New York: Recording & Statistical Company, 1964), 70–105.

51 See chapter 6 of my *Unnatural History: Breast Cancer and American Society* (Cambridge, U.K.: Cambridge University Press, 2007) for a similar story in cancer prevention, in which the post-WWII slogan became "every physician office a cancer detection center."

52 William Kannel, personal communication, May 1995. See Giroux, "Origines de l'étude prospective de cohorte," for a more complete discussion of this development.

53 E.g., H. A. Kahn, "A method for analyzing longitudinal observations on individuals in the Framingham heart study," *Proceedings of the Social Statistics Section, American Statistical Association* (Washington, D.C., American Statistical Association, 1961), 156–60. "Framingham pioneered progress in the use of statistical analysis to determine how risk factors are associated with disease," wrote William Castelli and William B. Kannel in 1987: "Risk factors for cardiovascular disease: the Framingham heart study," in *Forty Years of Achievement in Heart, Lung, and Blood Research* (Bethesda, Md., National Institutes of Health), 53–61, 56.

54 Thomas Dawber, personal communication, January 1997.

55 Other observers such as Sylvia Tesh have made the further criticism that multi-factorial theories of disease carry a hidden political agenda. In Tesh's view, multifactorial theories contribute to a pessimistic view of ever preventing chronic disease because of the difficulty of concerted action on all the multiple factors that would be required for change. They gain acceptance largely because they represent an ideologically appealing inertia and stupefaction about the causes of chronic disease. S. Tesh, *Hidden Arguments: Political Ideology and Disease Prevention Policy* (New Brunswick: Rutgers University Press, 1988).

56 Castelli and Kannel, "Risk factors for cardiovascular disease," 55.

57 H. Tunstall-Pedoe, "The Dundee coronary risk-disk for management of change in risk factors," *British Medical Journal*, 1991, 303 (6805): 744–47.

58 See, e.g., D. Moraes, P. McCormack, J. Tyrrell, and J. Feely, "Ear lobe crease and coronary heart disease," *Irish Medical Journal*, 1992, 85 (4): 131–32; W. J. Elliott, "Ear lobe crease and coronary artery disease: 1,000 patients and review of the literature," *American Journal of Medicine*, 1983, 75 (6): 1024–32; and E. Lichstein, K. D. Chadda, D. Naik, and P. K. Gupta, "Diagonal ear-lobe crease: prevalence and implications as a coronary risk factor," *New England Journal of Medicine*, 1974, 290 (11): 615–16. The literature on palm creases is much less substantial. See "The heart and the palm," *Time*, April 21, 1961, 64, for a lay report on such research. A. Keys, an early pioneer in CHD epidemiology, recognized the problematic aspects of the new statistical models, arguing that "the introduction of the multiple regression model, and its more elegant form in the multiple logistic equation, and the availability of computers and programs, allowed graduation from those earlier elementary analytic methods and the large loss of information they involved. That was a great step forward but it is not always appreciated that the analysis easily becomes a prisoner of the model." A. Keys, "From Naples to seven countries: a sentimental journey (epidemiological observations)," *Progress in Biochemical Pharmacology*, 1983, (19): 1–30, 14.

59 As a consequence of this endpoint problem, Kannel and others accepted that a large amount of the variance in the Framingham results was going to remain unexplained. This unsatisfying solution led others, such as the type A enthusiasts, to say that the risk factor mafia had missed two-thirds of the real causes, which in their view was due to a lack of interest in psychological states. See my *Making Sense of Illness: Science, Society, and Disease* (Cambridge, U.K.: Cambridge University Press, 1998), 145–65.

60 T. Dawber, W. Kannel, and L. Lyell, "An approach to longitudinal studies in a community: the Framingham study," *Annals of the New York Academy of Sciences*, 1963, 197: 539–56, 540.

61 E.g., "There is sometimes a tendency to regard an experiment as providing a higher form of evidence. This seems to us completely unrealistic." Gordon et al., "Some methodological problems in the long-term study of cardiovascular disease," 202.

62 T. R. Dawber and W. B. Kannel, "Susceptibility to coronary heart disease," *Modern Concepts of Cardiovascular Disease*, 1961, 30 (7): 671–76, 673.

63 E. Y. Brown, C. M. Viscoli, and R. I. Horwitz, "Preventive health strategies and the policy makers' paradox," *Annals of Internal Medicine*, 1992, 116 (7): 593–97.

64 William Kannel, personal communication, May 1995. In this section, I am focusing on the funding controversies in the late 1960s that resulted in Framingham's rebirth as an externally funded NIH project. There was a 1965 review, extensively and creatively explored by S. Patel ("Methods and management: NIH administrators, federal oversight, and the Framingham Heart

Study," *Bulletin of the History of Medicine*, 2012, 86 (1): 94–121), which initially led then NIH director James Shannon to seriously consider ending the study. Patel's analysis convincingly argues that the origin of this skepticism was a managerial style, steeped in the laboratory culture and priorities of most NIH administrators as well as in the rhetoric and politics of congressman and others charged with federal oversight of large NIH budgets, that emphasized tangible and predictable payoffs for money spent.

65 William Kannel, personal communication, May 1995.

66 Letter from Paul Dudley White to President Richard Nixon, dated September 2, 1969, in the Paul Dudley White Papers, Francis A. Countway Library of Medicine, Boston, HMS c36, box 37, folder 13.

67 William Kannel, personal communication, May 1995.

68 William Kannel, personal communication, May 1995.

69 Criticism of the risk factor approach as being too individualistic has come from many quarters, e.g., J. Cassel, "The contribution of the social environment to host resistance," *American Journal of Epidemiology*, 1976, 104 (2): 109; P. B. Peacock, "Health maintenance: a strategy for preventing cancer and heart disease," *Bulletin of the New York Academy of Medicine*, 1975, 51 (1): 100; and U. Goldbourt, "High risk versus public health strategies in primary prevention of coronary heart disease," *American Journal of Clinical Nutrition*, 1987, 45: 1185–92. Two later critiques that have become canonical for the emerging field of population health are G. Rose, "Sick individuals and sick populations," *International Journal of Epidemiology*, 1985, 14 (1): 32–38, and B. Link and J. C. Phelan, "Social conditions as fundamental causes of disease," *Journal of Health and Social Behavior*, 1995, 35: 80–94. See also Giroux, "Origines de l'étude prospective de cohorte," for an interesting contrast to contemporary British epidemiological approaches to CHD, which had a decidedly more "social medicine" approach, as well as discussion of the contrasting faith in the predictive meaning of "risk factors" between study investigators and Office of Biometry statisticians.

70 William Kannel, personal communication, May 1995.

71 Aronowitz, *Making Sense of Illness*.

72 There are so many instances in the Framingham study in which these practical, moral, and randomness-banishing functions of risk factors were revealed. Framingham investigators once dismissed the power of vitamin supplements to protect against CHD, by saying in effect that it is crazy to think that you can take a pill that would allow you to eat all the hamburgers you want without suffering cardiovascular consequences. W. B. Kannel and T. Thom, "Implications of the recent decline in cardiovascular mortality," *Cardiovascular Medicine*, 1979, 4: 983–97. In other words, there can be no simple escape from those dietary and behavioral choices that science has deemed bad. I have been witness to so many comments from both physician and nonphysician colleagues that it is not surprising when an obese, smoking, sedentary fifty-year-old male who has modestly elevated blood pressure and serum cholesterol should get a heart attack; in these casual comments and observations, the predictive "likely" blends imperceptibly with the "ought" of responsibility.

Chapter 5

1 This chapter has been modified from R. Aronowitz, "Gardasil: a vaccine against cancer and a drug to reduce risk," in *Three Shots at Prevention: The HPV Vaccine and the Politics of Medicine's Simple Solutions*, ed. K. Wailoo, J. Livingston,

S. Epstein, and R. Aronowitz, pp. 21–38. © 2010 The Johns Hopkins University Press. Reprinted with permission of the Johns Hopkins University Press.

2 www.youtube.com/watch?v=hJ8x3KR75fA, accessed January 11, 2008.

3 The advertisement is available at http://drflisser.com/flisserhpvcolposcopy .html, accessed January 11, 2008.

4 See G. Chesler and B. Kessler, "Re-presenting choice: tune in HPV," in K. Wailoo, J. Livingston, S. Epstein, and R. Aronowitz, eds., *Three Shots at Prevention: The HPV Vaccine and the Politics of Medicine's Simple Solutions* (Baltimore: Johns Hopkins University Press, 2010), 146–64. Controversies over vaccines have long been at the forefront of popular opposition to medicalization. They have also repeatedly ignited controversy over how benefit and risk are distributed; see J. Colgrove, *State of Immunity: The Politics of Vaccination in Twentieth-Century America* (Berkeley: University of California Press, 2006). In particular, vaccines have generally been given to healthy people at no special risk, often to children. Sometimes groups have borne risk only for the benefit of others (as in rubella vaccination for boys).

5 While vaccines have had positive effects on population health, mostly by herd immunity, they may also have deleterious population-level effects. The abandonment of smallpox vaccination, a consequence of the global eradication campaign's success, has led to population vulnerability to bioterrorism. Varicella vaccination, while reducing morbidity in childhood, is less effective than wild-type infection in producing immunity in the entire population. As a result, widespread immunization might lead to more susceptibility in adults, who are more likely to suffer serious disease. Other possible types of negative population impact include hyperreactivity (e.g., asthma) that may result from delayed exposure to infectious diseases because of mass vaccination and other phenomena (the so-called hygiene hypothesis) and the ecological changes in the type and virulence of infectious agents induced by vaccination's potential selection effects on wild-type infectious disease (considered in the section "'Scientific' efficacy of cervical cancer vaccines is uncertain").

6 L. Braun and L. Phoun, "HPV vaccination campaign: masking uncertainty, erasing complexity," in *Three Shots at Prevention*, 39–60.

7 P. Vineis and M. Berwick, "The population dynamics of cancer: a Darwinian perspective," *International Journal of Epidemiology*, 2006, 35 (5): 1151–59.

8 Testimony of Dr. Eliav Barr, minutes of FDA Center for Biologics Evaluation and Research, Vaccines and Related Biological Products Advisory Committee, November 28, 2001, p. 128.

9 Testimony of Laura Koutsky, who said that "we probably know more about the way HPV 16 and 18 cause cervical cancer than we know about how other agents cause other cancers." Ibid., 125.

10 See J. Cairns, *Matters of Life and Death: Perspectives on Public Health, Molecular Biology, Cancer, and the Prospects for the Human Race* (Princeton, NJ: Princeton University Press, 1997), especially 188–90.

11 Pap smears—which detect abnormal cells that might be indicative of cervical cancer or precancer—do not in themselves lead to any health benefit. Instead, they can trigger different types of treatment, such as cryosurgery, laser surgery, cone biopsies, hysterectomies, radiation, or more intense surveillance that later leads to treatment.

12 Although since the introduction of the polio vaccine in the 1950s we have had clinical trials of vaccines, at no time has the problem of evaluating efficacy and safety been easy. Clinical trials have not extinguished uncertainty or controversy. Even when done well, such trials must use limited endpoints and short time horizons. By chance alone, trials may produce putative evidence of benefit

and harm. Efficacy has been especially hard to evaluate at the population level, since many diseases are already declining for apparently nonspecific reasons related to socioeconomic advancement. It has also not helped contain controversy that so many "clinical trials" of vaccines were ad hoc experiments done on vulnerable populations such as prison inmates and institutionalized children.

13 While I find it highly likely that Pap smear screening has been effective at reducing cervical cancer mortality, other explanations for the larger secular trend are possible, e.g., rising hysterectomy rates in the post–World War II period.

14 C. Munoz-Almagro, I. Jordan, A. Gene, C. Latorre, J. J. Garcia-Garcia, and R. Pallares, "Emergence of invasive pneumococcal disease caused by non-vaccine serotypes in the era of 7-valent conjugate vaccine," *Clinical Infection Disease*, 2008, 46 (2): 174–82.

15 J. Greene, *Prescribing by Numbers: Drugs and the Definition of Disease* (Baltimore: Johns Hopkins University Press, 2006). This argument was presented in very similar form in R. Aronowitz, "Framing disease: an underappreciated mechanism for the social patterning of health," *Social Science and Medicine*, 2008, 67 (1): 1–9.

16 A. Brandt, "Blow some my way," *Clio Medicine* 46 (1998): 164–91.

17 Herschel Lawson, presenter, minutes of CDC National Immunization Program, Advisory Committee on Immunization Practices, June 29, 2005, p. 69, noted that an astounding 82 percent of U.S. women had a Pap test in the three years prior to 2000, according to the National Health Interview Survey and the Behavioral Risk Factor Surveillance System.

18 See my discussion of lobular carcinoma in situ and other embodied risks in R. Aronowitz, *Unnatural History: Breast Cancer and American Society* (Cambridge, U.K.: Cambridge University Press, 2007), 273–75.

19 See also the analysis of Merck's HPV "True Stories" website in chapter 3. Given these fears and concerns, I wondered why HPV risk was not given more medical or popular attention in recent years (until Merck's "tell someone" campaign), especially since wide media attention was given to genital herpes and HIV risk. One explanation, but one that itself needs some analysis, is the minor cultural visibility of cervical cancer and other HPV-related health problems, as evidenced and constituted by the lack of prominent cervical cancer lay advocacy groups.

20 For an insightful and textured analysis of the decision making with regard to cervical cancer vaccines, see J. A. Reich, "Parenting and prevention: views of HPV vaccines among parents challenging childhood immunizations," in *Three Shots at Prevention*, 165–81. In contrast to what is commonly said about parental concerns, for example, few parents in this study worried that the vaccine would encourage promiscuity or early sexual activity.

21 Coming close to explicitly selling fear are the "true story" videos on Merck's website, one of which I discussed in chapter 3.

22 www.youtube.com/watch?v=grVqRnDgS8w, accessed January 11, 2008.

23 www.youtube.com/watch?v=nsROPHTQzFE; accessed January 11, 2008.

24 See A. Leader, J. Weiner, C. Bigman, R. Hornik, and J. Cappella, "The effects of information framing on intentions to vaccinate against human papilloma virus" (abstract), Fifth AACR International Conference on Frontiers in Cancer Prevention Research, November 12–15, 2006, for some experimental evidence for lesser demand for a vaccine aimed at an STD and cancer rather than cancer alone.

25 A competing bivalent vaccine (16, 18) was also introduced in the American

market. The makers of this vaccine have made a different bet—that there might be fewer side effects and greater immunity to the two cancer-associated HPV types without the VLPs of other HPV types, as well as a different (AS04) adjuvant.

26 Galambos and Sewell observed that varicella vaccine was the last attenuated live-virus vaccine and hepatitis A vaccine the last killed-virus vaccine. L. Galambos and J. E. Sewell, *Networks of Innovation: Vaccine Development at Merck, Sharp and Dohme and Mulford, 1895–1995* (New York: Cambridge University Press, 1995), 235.

27 Lawson, in minutes of CDC, National Immunization Program, p. 70.

28 A similar kind of efficacy has attracted attention in prostate cancer prevention. A clinical experiment of Finasteride for the primary prevention of cancer had initially been understood as a negative trial. Cancers that were prevented were unlikely to cause harm while the group taking the drug had higher rates of more serious cancer. Longer and more complete follow-up dampened the latter association and allowed for a new interpretation of preventing benign disease. Finasteride led to much less unnecessary workup and treatment, saving money and iatrogenic harm. This benefit, however, would only be seen in a population of men undergoing PSA screening. See I. M. Thompson, P. J. Goodman, C. M. Tangen, H. L. Parnes, L. M. Minasian, P. A. Godley, M. S. Lucia, and L. G. Ford, "Long-term survival of participants in the prostate cancer prevention trial," *New England Journal of Medicine*, 2013, 369 (7): 603–10.

29 See the Digene HPV Test, at www.thehpvtest.com, accessed May 2, 2008.

30 G. Rose, "Sick individuals and sick populations," *International Journal of Epidemiology*, 1985, 14 (1): 32–38.

31 N. J. Wald and M. R. Law, "A strategy to reduce cardiovascular disease by more than 80%," *British Medical Journal*, 2003, 326: 1419–24.

32 Advertising and aggressive marketing of vaccines are not new phenomena. There was considerable social marketing of diphtheria vaccine. Merck was very active in marketing its measles vaccine. Nor is the backlash from different quarters about a drug company's overreaching in its manipulation of demand and the regulatory process in itself new to Gardasil. Colgrove documented the way excessive actions of Dow Chemical's promotion of its rubella vaccine led to a backlash against it (see his *State of Immunity*).

33 See chapter 8 and D. Ramogola-Masire, "Cervical cancer, HIV, and the HPV vaccine in Botswana," in *Three Shots at Prevention*, 91–102, which highlights the very different disease that any HPV vaccine will have to target in Africa and other resource-poor places. Not only is there a different prevalence of cancer-causing HPV serotypes, but coinfection with HIV (leading to greater numbers of affected women with more aggressive disease), nearly absent cervical cancer screening, and little attention to women's health complicate the picture.

Chapter 6

1 G. B. Shaw, *The Philanderer*, 1893. Available online at: http://www.gutenberg.org/catalog/world/readfile?fk_files=1458096.

2 R. Aronowitz, "Lyme disease: the social construction of a new disease, and its social consequences" *Milbank Quarterly*, 1991, 69: 79-112.

3 R. B. Stricker, A. Lautin, and J. J. Burrascano, "Lyme disease: point/counterpoint," *Expert Review of Anti-infective Therapy*, 2005, 3: 155–65.

4 G. P. Wormser, R. J. Dattwyler, E. D. Shapiro, J. J. Halperin, A. C. Steere, M. S. Klempner, P. J. Krause, J. S. Bakken, F. Strle, G. Stanek, L. Bockenstedt, D. Fish,

J. S. Dumler, and R. B. Nadelman, "The clinical assessment, treatment, and prevention of Lyme disease, human granulocytic anaplasmosis, and babesiosis: clinical practice guidelines by the Infectious Diseases Society of America," *Clinical Infectious Diseases*, 2006, 43: 1089–1134.

5 For a discussion of what appears to be at stake in these long-lasting controversies, see Aronowitz, "Lyme disease."

6 P. Murray, *The Widening Circle: A Lyme Disease Pioneer Tells Her Story* (New York: St. Martin's Press, 1996), 121.

7 For an insightful overview of these individuals and groups and the personal journey many LD patients follow, prompted by the limitations of existing knowledge and medical care, which lead them and their families to find other members—patients and doctors—of the heterodox community, see P. Weintraub, *Cure Unknown: Inside the Lyme Epidemic* (New York: St. Martin's Griffin, 2009).

8 L. H. Sigal, J. M. Zahradnik, P. Lavin, S. J. Patella, G. Bryant, R. Haselby, E. Hilton, M. Kunkel, D. Adler-Klein, T. Doherty, J. Evans, P. J. Molloy, A. L. Sidner, J. R. Sabetta, H. J. Simon, M. S. Klempner, J. Mays, D. Marks, and S. E. Malawista, "A vaccine consisting of recombinant *Borrelia burgdorferi* outer-surface protein A to prevent Lyme disease," *New England Journal of Medicine* 1998, 339: 216–22; A. C. Steere, V. K. Sikand, F. Meurice, D. L. Parenti, E. Fikrig, R. T. Schoen, J. Nowakowski, C. H. Schmid, S. Laukamp, C. Buscarino, and D. S. Krause. 1998. "Vaccination against Lyme disease with recombinant *Borrelia burgdorferi* outer-surface lipoprotein with adjuvant," *New England Journal of Medicine*, 1998, 339: 209–15.

9 L. Altman, "F.D.A. experts back a vaccine against lyme," *New York Times*, May 27, 1998, A1.

10 Chinh Le, 12. ACIP (Advisory Committee on Immunization Practices) of the Centers for Disease Control and Prevention, 1998, meeting minutes, June 24–25; available by request to Centers for Disease Control and Prevention.

11 David Denns, 12. ACIP meeting minutes, October 21, 1998.

12 Paul Offit, personal communication, June 2011.

13 Not unlike other pharmaceutical companies in the 1980s and 1990s, Connaught underwent rapid-fire changes in ownership and administration. The company's acquisition in 1990 by the Mérieux Institute (which had recently acquired Pasteur Production) for almost a billion dollars was widely reported as a sign that the hitherto moribund (in terms of profits) vaccine industry was entering a new era. The promise of a financially successful LD vaccine, which was already in the works at Connaught, was presumably part of this attraction. One article reported that Mérieux expected to increase its vaccine sales from $547 million in 1988 to $2.5 billion in 2000 (E. Andrews, "A major revival in research on vaccines," *New York Times*, August 22, 1990, D7).

14 Leonard Sigal, personal communication, July 2011.

15 Stanley Plotkin, personal communication, July 18, 2011.

16 Loren Cooper, personal communication, August 11, 2011.

17 A. Rierdan, "Testing for a Lyme disease vaccine," *New York Times*, December 1, 1996, CN1.

18 A. Steere, VRBPAC (Vaccines and Related Biological Products Advisory Committee) of the Food and Drug Administration, meeting minutes, May 26, 1998; available at http://www.fda.gov/ohrms/dockets/ac/98/transcpt/3422t1.pdf (accessed July 19, 2010). Although SKB merged with Glaxo Wellcome in 2000 to form GlaxoSmithKline, I will continue to refer to SKB in this period to preserve continuity.

19 VRBPAC (Vaccines and Related Biological Products Advisory Committee) of the Food and Drug Administration, meeting minutes, January 31, 2001; avail-

able at: http://www.fda.gov/ohrms/dockets/ac/01/transcripts/3680t2_01.pdf (accessed July 12, 2010).

20 S. Lurie, VRBPAC, meeting minutes, January 31, 2001.

21 B. Luft, VRBPAC, meeting minutes, January 31, 2001.

22 Loren Cooper, personal communication, August 11, 2011.

23 R. Schoen, VRBPAC, meeting minutes, May 26, 1998.

24 A. Barbour, "Let scientists do their job," *New York Times*, July 5, 1997, A23.

25 J. Colgrove, *State of Immunity: The Politics of Vaccination in Twentieth-Century America*. (Berkeley: University of California Press, 2006).

26 D. Snider, VRBPAC, meeting minutes, January 31, 2001.

27 P. Easton, VRBPAC, meeting minutes, January 31, 2001.

28 K. Vanderhoof-Forschner, VRBPAC, meeting minutes, January 31, 2001.

29 S. Jasanoff, *States of Knowledge: The Co-production of Science and the Social Order* (London: Routledge, 2006). D. Weld, VRBPAC, meeting minutes, May 26, 1998.

30 R. Daum, VRBPAC, meeting minutes, January 31, 2001.

31 M. Dixson, VRBPAC, meeting minutes, January 31, 2001.

32 K. Lyon, VRBPAC, meeting minutes, January 31, 2001.

33 K. Lyon, VRBPAC, meeting minutes. January 31, 2001.

34 P. Smith, VRBPAC, meeting minutes, January 31, 2001.

35 L. Gerlbert, VRBPAC, meeting minutes, January 31, 2001.

36 R. Neustadt and H. Fineberg, *The Swine Flu Affair: Decision-Making on a Slippery Disease* (Washington, D.C.: U.S. Department of Health, Education, and Welfare, 1978).

37 R. A. Kalish, M. Leong, and A. C. Steere, "Association of treatment-resistant chronic Lyme arthritis with HLA-DR4 and antibody reactivity of OspA and OspB of *Borrelia burgdorferi*," *Infection and Immunity*, 1993, 61 (7): 2774–79.

38 Leonard Sigal, personal communication, July 6, 2011.

39 D. France, "Lyme expert developed big picture of tiny tick," *New York Times*, May 4, 1999, F7.

40 K. Shea, "Glaxo settles Lyme disease vaccine suit," *Philadelphia Inquirer*, July 9, 2003, B3.

41 There were also claims of actual harm, some of which were settled by the company out of court to avoid the expense and uncertainty of litigation, according to SKB lawyers (Loren Cooper, personal communication, August 11, 2011).

42 J. Marra, VRBPAC, meeting minutes, January 31, 2001.

43 R. Aronowitz, *Making Sense of Illness: Science, Society, and Disease* (Cambridge, U.K.: Cambridge University Press, 1998).

44 For a general argument about the nexus of lay and scientific ideas about immunity in etiological thinking, see E. Martin, *Flexible Bodies* (Boston: Beacon Press, 1994). Asthma has perhaps only borderline status as an autoimmune process, as it has external triggers and is not a direct immune attack on "the self." Nevertheless, it is often included in this class of disorders and despite the external trigger, the end result is an exaggerated and unwanted inflammatory response.

45 Since I first drafted this essay, longer-term results from a clinical trial testing Finasteride's role in prostate cancer prevention have appeared that have shown interesting and confusing results—apparent decrease in early stage cancers but an increase in more deadly ones. There are multiple interpretations of both the causes and implications of these results. See I. M. Thompson, P. J. Goodman, C. M. Tangen, H. L. Parnes, L. M. Minasian, P. A. Godley, M. S. Lucia, and L. G. Ford, "Long-term survival of participants in the prostate cancer prevention trial," *New England Journal of Medicine*, 2013, 369 (7): 603–10.

46 H. G. Welch, L. Schwartz, and S. Woloshin, *Overdiagnosed: Making People Sick in the Pursuit of Health* (Boston: Beacon Press, 2011).

47 Direct bodily harm from cancer screening has occasionally played a role in controversies. In the 1970s, opposition to screening mammography erupted into public controversy largely because radiation risk from mammography was raised as a theoretical concern. R. Aronowitz, *Unnatural History: Breast Cancer and American Society* (Cambridge, U.K.: Cambridge University Press. 2007).

48 R. Platt, VRBPAC, meeting minutes, January 31, 2001.

49 S. Wolfe, VRBPAC, meeting minutes, January 31, 2001.

50 S. Plotkin, ACIP, meeting minutes, June 24–25, 1998.

51 D. Goetzl, "SmithKline readies DTC effort for Lyme disease vaccine," *Advertising Age* (online journal), April 17, 2000; available at http://adage.com/article/news/smithkline-readies-dtc-effort-lyme-disease-vaccine/58685/ (accessed July 7, 2011).

52 Available at http://www.newspaperarchive.com/SiteMap/FreePdfPreview.aspx?img=149837946.

53 Leonard Sigal (personal communication, July 6, 2011) did not think the DTCA campaign was a major cause of LD fear. Instead, he blamed infusion companies who sponsored billboards encouraging fears of Lyme disease and including telephone numbers to operators who referred people to "Lyme literate" practitioners.

54 See previous chapter.

55 A. Revkin, "2 firms seeking approval of Lyme disease vaccines," *New York Times*, February 4, 1997, B4.

56 Both enthusiasm and apprehension could have been read into what had transpired earlier in the decade with dog LD vaccines. A *New York Times* article reported that "with the aid of aggressive marketing, the [dog] vaccine found a ready public. Since last July nearly two million doses have been sold" (E. Eckholm, "Caution is urged on Lyme disease vaccinations for dogs," *New York Times*, June 22, 1991, 48). But there was a backlash to the successful, aggressive marketing. Organized veterinarians and the U.S. Department of Agriculture urged that the vaccine be limited to dogs that were at high risk. They also voiced concerns that the dog vaccine might cause Lyme disease–like symptoms. Another account of dog vaccine backlash reported that Alan Barbour, a codiscoverer of *B. burgdorferi*, had seen a billboard in Houston, where there was no LD risk, which queried "Has your dog been vaccinated for Lyme?" (R. Weiss, "Vaccine trial begins against Lyme disease, *Washington Post* June 21, 1994, F7).

57 A. Steere, "Lyme borreliosis in 2005, 30 years after initial observations in Lyme, Connecticut," *Wiener klinische Wochenschrift*, 2006, 118 (21–22): 625–33.

58 Leonard Sigal, personal communication, July 6, 2011; Paul Offit, personal communication, June 28, 2011; Stanley Plotkin, personal communication, July 18, 2011.

59 Backlash and distrust of pharmaceutical promotion was present throughout the brief history of these vaccines. When SKB announced at the end of the pre-marketing trial that it was giving the vaccine to the 5,000 participants who had been in the placebo arm, there was an immediate backlash (Revkin, "2 firms seeking approval of Lyme disease vaccines") by critics arguing that this was an empty marketing gesture designed to excite the investment community, not to improve anyone's health.

60 Aronowitz, "Lyme disease."

61 S. Epstein, *Impure Science: AIDS, Activism, and the Politics of Knowledge* (Berkeley: University of California Press, 1996).

62 S. Epstein, *Inclusion: The Politics of Difference in Medical Research*, (Chicago: University of Chicago Press, 2007).

63 S. Wolfe, VRBPAC, meeting minutes, January 31, 2001.

Chapter 7

1   S. Reuben, *Living Beyond Cancer: A European Dialogue*, President's Cancer Panel, 2003–2004 Annual Report, May 2004; accessed May 2011 at http://deainfo .nci.nih.gov/advisory/pcp/annualReports/pcp03-04rpt/Supplement.pdf. Despite this important usage difference, the term *survivor* is used in almost every paragraph of this forty-plus page report (written in English).

2   M. Markman, "Cancer survivorship: the concept and the increasingly recognized reality," *Current Oncology Reports*, 2006, 8 (2): 79–80.

3   Text search using the term "cancer survivor" in the historical database of the *New York Times* from 1900 to 2007.

4   W. Kaempffert, "Science in review: some papers of special interest among the 400 read before Medical Association," *New York Times*, June 7, 1953, E11.

5   The graphic representation of this cohort experience is the survival or Kaplan–Meier curve, named after the statisticians who developed it.

6   T. Lasser, *Reach to Recovery* (New York: Simon and Schuster, 1972).

7   J. Klemesrud, "Those who have been there aid breast surgery patients," *New York Times*, February 8, 1971, 28.

8   "An individual is considered a cancer survivor from the time of diagnosis, through the balance of his or her life. Family members, friends, and caregivers are also impacted by the survivorship experience and are therefore included in this definition." R. Twombly, "What's in a name: who is a cancer survivor?" *Journal of the National Cancer Institute*, 2004, 96 (19): 1414–15.

9   Centers for Disease Control, "Cancer Survivorship—United States, 1971–2001," *MMWR*, 2004, 53(24): 526–29.

10 http://www.cancer.gov/newscenter/pressreleases/2011/survivorshipMMWR 2011; accessed July 2011.

11 R. Aronowitz, *Unnatural History: Breast Cancer and American Society* (Cambridge, U.K.: Cambridge University Press, 2007).

12 H. G. Welch, L. Schwartz, and S. Woloshin, *Overdiagnosed: Making People Sick in the Pursuit of Health* (Boston: Beacon Press, 2011).

13 Cancer survivorship is also consistent with an American "therapeutic culture." For example, Paul Rabinow describes how the experience of trauma has defined new syndromes, e.g., incest survivors. P. Rabinow, "Artificiality and enlightenment: from sociobiology to biosociality," *Essays on the Anthropology of Reason* (Princeton, NJ: Princeton University Press, 1996).

14 http://www.seer.cancer.gov/statfacts/html/lungb.html#incidence-mortality. accessed July 2011. The spectrum of lung cancer cases may soon change, however. Calls for screening smokers with spiral CT scans may lead to the kind of diagnostic expansion that happened in breast and prostate cancer, i.e. the diagnosis and treatment of cancers whose malignant potential is low.

15 A. L. Buscher and T. P. Giordano, "Gaps in knowledge in caring for HIV survivors long-term," *Journal of the American Medical Association*, 2010, 304 (3): 340–41.

16 http://community.breastcancer.org/forum/68/topic/756781; accessed July 2011.

17 I have observed that few people allow themselves to question the decision to

have extensive treatment for DCIS and other borderline risk/cancer diagnoses either on the basis of more definitive pathology, their own posttreatment cancer-free lives, or new aggregate data and/or interpretations of such data. While I am reticent to posit unobservable psychological motivations, the cognitive dissonance of doubting the ontological status of a cancer diagnosis while living with a decision for extensive treatment is great.

18 http://community.breastcancer.org/forum/68/topic/756781.

19 Aronowitz, *Unnatural History*.

20 Aronowitz, *Unnatural History*.

21 T. Lewin, "Changing view of cancer: something to live with," *New York Times*, February 4, 1991, A1.

22 F. Mullan, "Seasons of survival: reflections of a physician with cancer," *New England Journal of Medicine*, 1985, 313 (4): 270–73.

23 Some cancer regimens leave people posttreatment in need of continuous therapy, e.g., patients after stem cell transplant for acute myeloid leukemia often require continuous antirejection and anti-graft-vs.-host treatment.

24 The survivorship movement may lead to new forms of stigma and controversy, e.g., when people recruited into groups with titles like "living with" or "living beyond" one or another cancer discover that these groups are sometimes funded by and advance the cause of pharmaceutical companies and other narrow interests. These interests are motivated to build markets for present and future products. Survivors may feel duped and manipulated and become the object of their own or others' derision.

25 See for example L. M. Hoskins, K. M. Roy, and M. H. Greene, "Toward a new understanding of risk perception among young female BRCA1/2 'previvors,'" *Families, Systems, & Health*, 2012, 30 (1): 32–46.

26 For example, see http://www.survivorshipguidelines.org/pdf/ltfuguidelines.pdf, accessed December 28, 2014.

27 Physicians made such observations in online response to a *New England Journal of Medicine* clinical vignette of good-prognosis prostate cancer, which was followed by rationales for surgery, radiation, and watchful waiting. Online comments by survey participants can be viewed on http://proxy.library.upenn.edu:2253/clinical-decisions/20081211/#commentbox. A summary of the results was published in the journal itself: R. S. Schwartz, "Management of prostate cancer—polling results," *New England Journal of Medicine*, 2009, 360: e4.

28 See chapter 3 for full discussion of what am calling "social efficacy." The standard historical reference for this way of understanding efficacy remains C. Rosenberg, "The therapeutic revolution: Medicine, meaning, and social change in nineteenth-century America," *Perspectives in Biology and Medicine*, 1977, 20 (4): 485–506.

29 The same term is not used in Hebrew to denote the person who outlives cancer and the Holocaust.

30 B. Bettelheim, *Surviving & Other Essays* (New York: Alfred A. Knopf, 1979).

31 Many other critics have observed the inappropriate optimism, mindless positivity, and kitschy feminine stereotypes of some breast cancer awareness and (often big pharma–funded) activism, as well as their problematic alliances with drug companies. See, for example, B. Ehrenreich, "Welcome to Cancerland: a mammogram leads to a cult of pink kitsch," *Harper's Magazine*, November 2001, 43–53, and S. King, *Pink Ribbons, Inc.: Breast Cancer and the Politics of Philanthropy* (Minneapolis: University of Minnesota Press, 2006).

32 S. L. Jain, "Living in prognosis: toward an elegiac politics," *Representations*, 2007, 98: 77–92.

33 Advertisement for Greenwich Hospital in *New York Times*, March 20, 1994, 8.
34 Advertisement for talk at Cancer Center at Hackensack Hospital, *New York Times*, June 13, 1993, D9.
35 R. C. Rabin, "A pink ribbon race, years long," *New York Times*, January 17, 2011, D1.
36 Rabin, "A pink ribbon race, years long."

Chapter 8

1 The Indian pharmaceutical industry has been rapidly expanding, driven in part by global demand and changes to patent laws that have encouraged domestic production of drugs still under patent elsewhere. Bode has documented how even traditional Ayurvedic medicines have expanded and morphed into commodities via Western marketing practices. And vice versa—Vicks VapoRub has been classified as an "Ayurvedic proprietary medicine," which among other things gets favorable tax treatment under Indian law. M. Bode, "Taking traditional knowledge to the market: the commoditization of Indian medicine," *Anthropology & Medicine*, 2006, 13 (3): 225–36.

2 S. R. Whyte, S. van der Geest, and A. Hardon, *Social Lives of Medicines* (Cambridge, U.K.: Cambridge University Press, 2002).

3 In 1988 there were other harbingers of change. There were no definitive HIV-AIDS cases in our hospital, almost certainty due to the lack of resources with which to diagnose HIV and most opportunistic infections. But there were cases like a previously healthy young man who quickly developed life-threatening pulmonary tuberculosis. He almost certainly was suffering from HIV/AIDS.

4 While I have had little direct involvement in what has come to be known as global health, there are seemingly daily reminders that public health, clinical, and consumer practices have complex provenances and global reach and interactions, e.g., the geographically spread-out populations of research subjects cited in methods sections of clinical studies or newspaper coverage of manufacturing scandals of prescription and over-the-counter medicines in faraway places.

5 There have, of course, been examples of consumer health products exported from rich to poor regions that posed health risks and were recognized as such and led to local opposition and global controversy, e.g., Nestle's aggressive marketing of infant formula to poor countries that led to a worldwide boycott of the company's products.

6 See J. Livingston, B. Cooper, and K. Wailoo, "HPV skepticism and vaccination as governance: the U.S. and Africa as a lens onto the north-south divide," in *Three Shots at Prevention: The HPV Vaccine and the Politics of Medicine's Simple Solutions*, ed. K. Wailoo, J. Livingston, S. Epstein, and R. Aronowitz (Baltimore: Johns Hopkins University Press, 2010). Risk-reducing practices such as HPV vaccination and cervical cancer screening have complicated multifocal origins, e.g., some of the basic insights about the HPV-cancer link and vaccine structure were made in Germany and Australia, and clinical trials of early vaccines were done in sites all over the world. Similarly with cervical cancer screening, there has been considerable variation, innovation, and cross-fertilization among North American and European countries. See, especially, Ilana Lowy's comparative work in cervical cancer, *A Woman's Disease: The History of Cervical Cancer* (Oxford: Oxford University Press, 2011) and *Prevention Strikes: Women, Precancer, and Prophylactic Surgery* (Baltimore: Johns Hopkins University Press, 2010). Evaluating the efficacy of screening programs presents special problems.

Screening itself typically has no direct effect on health. Instead, efficacy results from things screening triggers, such as medicines or surgery. Effects—positive and negative—are usually small and often difficult to measure and perceive. These are permissive conditions for the fierce debates over the interpretation of evidence for screening mammography and PSA testing that have erupted in the U.S. and other developed countries. These problems are only compounded in poor countries where there are generally fewer resources for surveillance and evaluation.

7 Some risk-reducing practices and products have perhaps more potential to cause overtreatment in poorer countries or among the poorer segments of middle-income and rich countries. For example, the *New England Journal of Medicine* recently conducted an online poll of its readership about the best treatment of a hypothetical patient with early good-prognosis prostate cancer (although not indicated, this clinical dilemma is most often the result of cancer screening). The readership was roughly equally divided among watchful waiting, surgery, and radiation. A few respondents from poor countries explained that they were choosing surgery over watchful waiting because their health systems did not have the technology to survey untreated patients for early signs of progression. Therefore, in underresourced settings, it made more sense to choose aggressive therapy. In addition, less extreme but more costly or technologically more complex interventions might not be available. For example, some doctors from non-Western countries explained that they felt compelled to do orchiectomies to treat prostate cancer recurrence because of the unavailability of hormonal treatment. R. S. Schwartz, "Clinical decisions. Management of prostate cancer—polling results," *New England Journal of Medicine*, January 1, 2009, 360 (3): e4.

8 Some of these concerns are subsumed within anthropological critiques, especially those that have extended Foucaultian notions of biopower to contemporary global health conditions by developing concepts such as biological and therapeutic citizenship. In the dysfunctional and ravaged Soviet and post-Soviet Ukraine, Petryna deployed *biological citizenship* to describe how claims of entitlement resulting from exposure to the nuclear accident at Chernobyl were used to negotiate rights, compensation, and recognition. The idiosyncrasy of individual suffering and the complexities of causal association have allowed individuals and groups to challenge political and scientific authority and make claims for legitimacy and compensation. At the same time, the bodily harm associated with exposure to catastrophic technological failure is a problematic basis for political rights, ensuring social justice, and sustaining democracy, while introducing distortions into the workings of health care. See A. Petryna, *Life Exposed: Biological Citizens after Chernobyl* (Princeton: Princeton University Press, 2002). Similarly, in the context of antiretroviral treatment for AIDS in Africa, Nguyen et al. proposed extending biopower and biological citizenship to *therapeutic* citizenship, which they defined as "claims made on a global social order on the basis of a therapeutic predicament." See V. Nguyen, C. Y. Ako, and P. Niamba, "Adherence as therapeutic citizenship: impact of the history of access to antiretroviral drugs on adherence to treatment," *AIDS*, 2007, 21:S1–S4. Nguyen and colleagues argue that by reducing individuals to their disease and their need for treatment, such practices exclude others who cannot make such claims, as well as distorting the needs and priorities of these same individuals besides therapeutic ones. At the same time, the near exclusive focus on providing HIV treatment can shift power to NGOs and other nonrepresentative groups for setting priorities and controlling the flow of resources.

9 Despite the problems of exporting existing HPV vaccines to poor countries,

deploying them is certainly a very good thing. This baby/bathwater problem recurs in many critical studies of global public health. Biehl studied antiretroviral treatment practices in Brazil, and acknowledged its many progressive features and effectiveness in saving lives. He nevertheless pointed out the resulting *pharmaceuticalization* of public health, in which individual-focused, medicalized interventions supplant more community-based ones. Biehl also argued that these programs may not always reach the most marginal people in a society and thus may contribute to their invisibility. J. Biehl, "Pharmaceutical governance," in *Global Pharmaceuticals: Ethics, Markets, Practices,* ed. A. Petryna, A. Lakoff, and A. Kleinman (Durham: Duke University Press, 2006).

10   http://www.cancer.gov/cancertopics/types/cervical, accessed April 2010.

11   In 2007–8, lifetime black/white chances of developing invasive cervical cancer and death from the disease were .94/.69 and .39/.22. http://www.cancer.org /downloads/STT/CAFF2007AAacspdf2007.pdf, facts and figures, accessed April 2010.

12   See summaries at http://info.cancerresearchuk.org/cancerstats/types/cervix /incidence/ and http://info.cancerresearchuk.org/cancerstats/types/cervix /mortality/, accessed April 2010. For a brilliant historical and ethnographic account of cervical (and other) cancer in Botswana, see J. Livingston, *Improvising Medicine: An African Oncology Ward in an Emerging Cancer Epidemic* (Durham: Duke University Press, 2012).

13   Gardasil contains two additional HPV VLPs targeted at preventing warts.

14   In the intervening years, there have been significant efforts to develop vaccines that cover more HPV types. Reports in the medical literature cite early-phase trials of second-generation vaccines that not only target more HPV types, but are cheaper to produce and may be orally administered, leading to greater possibilities for use in resource-poor regions. See S. Kiatpongsan, N. G. Campos, and J. J. Kim, "Potential benefits of second-generation human papillomavirus vaccines," *PLoS ONE,* 2012, 7 (11): e48426, http://www.plosone.org/article /info%3Adoi%2F10.1371%2Fjournal.pone.0048426#pone.0048426-Clinical TrialsGov1.

15   S. E. Powell, S. Hariri, M. Steinau, H. M. Bauer, N. M. Bennett, K. C. Bloch, L. M. Niccolai, S. Schafer, E. R. Unger, and L. E. Markowitz, "Impact of human papillomavirus (HPV) vaccination on HPV 16/18–related prevalence in precancerous cervical lesions," *Vaccine,* 2012, 31 (1): 109–13. Given the small numbers of expected cancer deaths and the long interval in which cancers develop, the clinical trials that initially established the vaccines' efficacy had to use intermediate measures such as reduced numbers of HPV-specific high-grade lesions, not mortality, as endpoints.

16   There is also hope that the existing vaccines provide some cross-reactivity against nontargeted HPV types, especially HPV 45.

17   The issue of greater patent protection for products produced by recombinant DNA technology has received renewed attention because of the Affordable Care Act. See A. So and S. Katz, "Biologics boondoggle," *New York Times,* Op-Ed, A23, March 9, 2010.

18   See for example, http://www.gardasilaccessprogram.org/section/141, accessed April 2010. According to the website, "The GARDASIL® Access Program will provide GARDASIL® to programs in eligible countries to allow countries to gain experience in the implementation of such programs. It does not aim to cover nationwide HPV vaccine programs. The program will draw upon the learnings and experiences from participating organizations and seek to con-

tribute to knowledge on how to successfully implement HPV vaccine access programs in developing countries." The access program noted Merck's earlier provision of Mectizan treatments against river blindness, which was the prototypical humanitarian medical intervention for the company. "We've been involved in a number of public-private partnerships in least developed countries to help make our products available for more than 20 years. Through the Merck Mectizan Donation Program we have donated more than 2.5 billion tablets of Mectizan for river blindness, with more than 700 million treatments approved since 1987. The program currently reaches more than 80 million people in Africa, Latin America and Yemen annually."

19 "For a business to succeed we must make profits in a way that is socially responsible, environmentally sustainable and politically acceptable," argued a Merck corporate responsibility (CR) officer. "If not, we will lose our implicit 'license to operate' from the public or lose out to the competition." http://www .gardasilaccessprogram.org/section/141, accessed April 2010. In the U.S., Merck's reputation as a moral firm has been eroded by the Vioxx debacle in the mid-2000s as well as the controversy that erupted over its heavy-handed manipulation of state-level policy making in support of Gardasil. Vaccine giveaway programs do something to keep these criticisms at bay while sustaining credibility and trust.

20 N. Muñoz, F. X. Bosch, X. Castellsagué, M. Díaz, S. de Sanjose, D. Hammouda, K. V. Shah, and C. J. Meijer, "Against which human papilloma virus types shall we vaccinate and screen? The international perspective," *International Journal of Cancer*, 2004, 111: 278–85. See also Livingston, *Improvising Medicine*, 44–45, for a more recent review of our uncertainties about HPV-cancer links in Africa. See also note 14 for more recent developments of oral vaccines that target nine HPV types.

21 J. Cohen, "Public health: high hopes and dilemmas for a cervical cancer vaccine," *Science*, 2005, 308 (5722): 618–21.

22 Cohen, "Public health."

23 A frequently observed example of this path dependency is the long persistence of the QWERTY keyboard.

24 An Indian newspaper account criticized HPV vaccination promoters in India on other grounds, including oversimplifying the complexity and efficacy of vaccines and cervical cancer prevention; giving the vaccine to girls after sexual exposure, when they are likely too late; and inadequate surveillance for vaccine side effects. R. Bhatia: "Vaccine no guarantee against cervical cancer," *India Times*, December 29, 2009, http://indiatoday.intoday.in/site/Story/76944 /Lifestyle/Vaccine+no+guarantee+against+cervical+cancer.html.

25 Department-Related Parliamentary Standing Committee on Health and Family Welfare, *Alleged Irregularities in the Conduct of Studies Using Human Papilloma Virus (HPV) Vaccine by PATH in India*, August 30, 2013, http://www.pharma medtechbi.com/~/media/Supporting%20Documents/Pharmasia%20News /2013/September/HPV%20Vaccines%20Parliameetnary%20Report%20%20 Aug%2031%202013.pdf; accessed December 2013.

26 http://www.thehindu.com/opinion/editorial/collusion-of-the-worst-kind /article5117415.ece; accessed April 4, 2014.

27 The Indian pharmaceutical industry is itself very large and global, with its own diverse and often aggressive business practices (see discussion below of Januvia), and is also highly interconnected with industries that originated in the U.S. and Europe. In this discussion of the HPV controversy, I am focusing on the largely U.S.-to-India movement of HPV vaccines and practices that is

occurring within a large and prominent NGO-directed global program. I do not want to suggest, however, that this traffic in health products, practices, and ideas is only or even typically unidirectional. In order to focus on the problematic consequences of the global circulation of practices, I am also minimizing the diversity of business and public practices within India and within Western countries.

28 See, for example, http://www.theguardian.com/global-development/2013 /oct/08/anti-hpv-vaccine-campaigners-cervical-cancer, accessed in April 2014.

29 Department-Related Parliamentary Standing Committee, *Alleged Irregularities*, 9.

30 Department-Related Parliamentary Standing Committee, *Alleged Irregularities*, 12.

31 Department-Related Parliamentary Standing Committee, *Alleged Irregularities*, 14.

32 Department-Related Parliamentary Standing Committee, *Alleged Irregularities*, p. 9 and elsewhere.

33 This toehold was almost upended as a result of Indian generic copying of Januvia and Merck's combination drug that combined Metformin with Januvia. Signaling perhaps the emerging importance of protecting drug patent rights for Indian's own burgeoning industry, Indian courts recently offered opinions protecting Merck's patent rights within India.

34 See J. Greene, *Prescribing by Numbers: Drugs and the Definition of Disease* (Baltimore: Johns Hopkins University Press, 2006), and J. Dumit, *Drugs for Life: How Pharmaceutical Companies Define Our Health* (Durham, NC: Duke University Press, 2012). The story of risk factor intervention against chronic disease in developed regions may be recapitulating itself in developing countries, especially those with growing middle classes and their purchasing power. According to a corporate responsibility officer at Merck, "Traditionally we have generated the majority of our revenues in developed markets, such as the U.S. and Western Europe. This is changing as pricing pressures in traditional markets squeeze profits. At the same time, in emerging markets such as China, India, Brazil and Russia, we are starting to see increased purchasing power as middle classes emerge and as governments invest more in the health of their citizens. We also are seeing a shift in prevalence of disease from infectious to chronic disease in these markets." http://www.gardasilaccessprogram.org/section/141, accessed April 2010. As pointed out above, pharmaceutical companies are not merely seeing a shift but promoting it.

35 "As part of its new commercial model (that moved away from the traditional commercial model in the pharmaceutical industry), Merck focused on more targeted communication to doctors through its reps, e-detailing and video detailing. It made extensive use of new media such as the Internet. Experts hailed Merck's marketing acumen and said that more companies were expected to follow a similar model in the future." http://www.icmrindia.org/CaseStudies /catalogue/Marketing/Merck%20New%20Product%20Development-Launch %20Strategy-Januvia.htm; accessed January 2, 2009. In the U.S., Merck has also marketed Januvia directly to consumers.

36 Very intensive and advanced diabetes care is of course available in India in high-tech hospitals and clinics that serve a richer clientele. See, for example, the website of a fee-for-service (with sliding scale) proprietary diabetes hospital in India: http://www.mvdiabetes.com/facilities.htm; accessed June 2014.

37 See Greene, *Prescribing by Numbers*, and H. M. Marks, *The Progress of Experiment: Science and Therapeutic Reform in the United States, 1900–1990* (Cambridge, U.K.: Cambridge University Press, 1997). In the week I first drafted

this chapter, there were new reports of the problematic safety and efficacy of another global blockbuster diabetes drug, Rosiglitazone (G. Harris, "Research ties diabetes drug to heart woes," *New York Times*, February 19, 2010) In recent years, there has been increasing concern about Januvia and its class of insulin inhibitors to cause pancreatic cancer; see http://www.nytimes.com/2013/05/31 /business/a-doctor-raises-questions-about-a-diabetes-drug.html; accessed December 2013.

38 The dangers of new medications do not simply need a long time to be recognized but are often new phenomena, resulting from medications being used on patients different from those tested, in different doses and modes of administration, and in novel combinations with other interventions. R. Aronowitz, "The social and economic influences on medication use and misuse," *Journal of General Internal Medicine*, 2012, 27(12): 1580–81.

39 Indian physicians have voiced almost all of these points; see http://apothecurry .wordpress.com/2009/11/12/januvia-and-galvus-a-different-take/; accessed January 2010. "A very senior drug safety expert based in New Delhi seemed rather disturbed by the popularity of these medicines. He felt it was alarming that two new drugs with a safety and efficacy track record that is still being established in clinical practice should be so well-received by the medical community. He also believed that in the absence of a pharmaco-vigilance system in India that keeps tabs on drug side-effects, doctors will know little about the side-effects that may surface once the drugs are widely-marketed."

40 These details are from J. Schwartz, "The first rotavirus vaccine and the politics of acceptable risk," *Milbank Quarterly* 2012, 90 (2): 278–310. Another rotavirus vaccine later cleared U.S. regulatory review and has been used globally.

41 P. Farmer, *Infections and Inequalities* (Berkeley: University of California Press, 1999).

42 A. W. Crosby, *The Columbian Exchange: Biological and Cultural Consequences of 1492* (Westport, CT: Greenwood Pub., 2003), W. H. McNeill, *Plagues and People* (New York: Anchor Press, 1976); J. Diamond, *Guns, Germs, and Steel: The Fates of Human Societies* (New York: Norton, 1999). These accounts (which are so wide-angled that they sometimes flatten out important details), however, do not emphasize the ways that the impact of infectious disease on colonized populations was compromised by the exercise of power by colonial conquerors, especially by undermining indigenous environmental and disease control practices. Steve Feierman, personal communication, August 2013; see also N. D. Cook, *Demographic Collapse: Indian Peru, 1520–1620* (Cambridge, U.K.: Cambridge University Press, 2004).

43 B. G. Link and J. Phelan, "Social conditions as fundamental causes of disease," *Journal of Health and Social Behavior*, 1995, extra issue, 80–94. In addition to the important points made by Link and Phelan, when it comes to health problems emanating from consumption, producers will find ways to eventually try to push products and patterns of consumption to the largest possible market, which often means further democratization/expansion of risk. At the same time, poorer people have fewer protections.

44 There is now a great deal of concern and speculation that while developed, industrialized countries contribute more to global warming, the negative consequences will be greater for poor countries.

45 A. Brandt, *The Cigarette Century: The Rise, Fall, and Deadly Persistence of the Product That Defined America* (New York: Basic Books, 2007).

46 J. A. Greene, "Making medicines essential: the evolving role of pharmaceuticals in global health," *BioSocieties* 2011, 6: 10–33.

47 The efforts of the Bill and Melinda Gates Foundation to improve global health

have been widely lauded but have not escaped criticism either. The foundation has been criticized for its overemphasis on technological solutions and the resulting distortion of local health priorities and social determinants of health. See D. McCoy, G. Kembhavi, J. Patel, and A. Luinte, "The Bill & Melinda Gates Foundation's grant-making programme for global health," *Lancet*, 2009, 373 (9675): 1645–53.

48   A conference organized by the Open Society on the state of cervical cancer screening and treatment in Eastern Europe for its grantees illustrates that the diverse and region-specific challenges to any singular global public health norm or goal. In the borderland regions of the former U.S.S.R., there were diverse practices and obstacles, resulting in incomplete—from the perspective of norms in the U.S.—uptake of Pap screening and gynecological follow-up, as well as the problem of overutilization. In Armenia, biopsies were done without colposcopy, impacting accuracy; in Georgia, too many women under thirty were using the screening system, going against recommendations to screen older women and using up limited resources; in Kazakhstan, there was no screening and "cervical cancer prevention is not a Ministry priority at this time." In peripheral Russia (Sakhalin), potentially effective preventive exams in the workplace from the Soviet era were not continued after the demise of the U.S.S.R. V. D. Tsua and A. E. Pollack, "Preventing cervical cancer in low-resource settings: how far have we come and what does the future hold?" *International Journal of Gynecology and Obstetrics*, 2005, 89: S55–S59. Of course, there is considerable diversity within Europe and the U.S. vis-à-vis cervical cancer screening and treatment. See Löwy, *Preventive Strikes*, for a historical perspective on comparative cervical cancer practices in the U.S. and France; and for differences in HPV vaccine practices and policy within Europe and the U.S., see I. Löwy, "HPV vaccination in context: a view from France," 270–92, and A. Stockl, "Public discourses and policymaking: the HPV vaccination from the European perspective," 254–69, both in K. Wailoo, J. Livingston, S. Epstein, and R. Aronowitz, eds., *Three Shots at Prevention: The HPV Vaccine and the Politics of Medicine's Simple Solutions* (Baltimore: Johns Hopkins University Press, 2010).

49   "Cytology is a subjective test and in programs without quality control/quality assurance it is virtually impossible to achieve and maintain the clinical performance of cytology. Cytology is labor intensive and to date has been refractory to high-throughput automated screening. Despite the low cost of consumables and because of the three reasons cited above, high-quality cytology is expensive in absolute terms and may not necessarily be the most cost-effective option for screening." S. J. Goldie, L. Gaffikin, J. D. Goldhaber-Fiebert, A. Gordillo-Tobar, C. Levin, C. Mahe, and T. C. Wright, "Cost-effectiveness of cervical-cancer screening in five developing countries," *New England Journal of Medicine*, 2005, 353 (20): 2158–68.

50   Lost in the controversies over cervical cancer prevention is the reality that *treatment* of cervical cancer in poor parts of the world is rare and challenging. Julie Livingston has studied the efforts of physicians and nurses to treat cervical (and other) cancers in Botswana, which has one of the highest standards of living and least amount of economic inequality in Africa. Livingston documented the extremely advanced disease at which patients present to medical care and the improvised diagnostic and therapeutic response. See Livingston, *Improvising Medicine*.

51   The argument is sometimes made that it makes little sense to use individualized clinical practices like Pap smears or DNA testing in poor regions because they are too expensive and divert resources from more effective practices and

policies, especially the upstream social, economic, and political determinants of population health. Paul Farmer characterizes such anti-medical-care and anti-technology beliefs as Luddite, and emphasizes some unfair and harmful implications for poor societies. Putting aside questions of justice, Farmer and others argue that health care and socioeconomic development do not constitute a zero-sum game. Not only is a population with adequate health care a healthy and thus more productive society, but medical care creates solidarity and trust, prerequisites for effective social and political change, including successful prevention and population health interventions. Farmer, *Infections and Inequalities*.

52 R. Sankaranarayanan, B. Nene, S. Shastri, K. Jayant, R. Muwonge, A. Budukh, S. Hingmire, S. G. Malvi, R. Thorat, A. Kothari, R. Chinoy, R. Kelkar, S. Kane, S. Desai, V. R. Keskar, R. Rajeshwarkar, N. Panse, and K. A. Dinshaw, "HPV screening for cervical cancer in rural India," *New England Journal of Medicine*, 2009, 360: 1385–94.

53 Current HPV DNA tests require at least seven hours for results to become available. More rapid HPV tests are now being developed so that the HPV DNA test may someday be as convenient to use as the older, simpler "see and treat" technologies.

54 The major effort to promote acetic acid- and cytology-based "see and treat" strategies in India and elsewhere continued undeterred, at least in the short term, by the lack of demonstrated efficacy in the *New England Journal of Medicine* report. A fact sheet from the ACCP argued that one study alone, no matter how well done, should not trump earlier studies that showed that direct visualization with simple stains followed by cryotherapy was effective. The ACCP argued that these low-tech approaches were simpler, cheaper, efficacious, and much easier to deploy in poor countries. Moreover, existing low-tech "see and treat" programs have been key to establishing community education and sensitization and greater awareness of cervical cancer, i.e., these practices had other important efficacies besides saving lives from cervical cancer. They also argued that "see and treat" programs will remain "an important component of an HPV DNA test-based program, as it is used to triage women who should not receive cryotherapy due to large lesions or suspected cancer." http://www.rho.org/files/ACCP_screening_factsheet_July09.pdf; accessed 4 April 2010.

55 There are other acknowledged problems with "see and treat" strategies mentioned in the scientific literature and news reports: What does this program mean for women and health care workers on the ground? What are the indirect and ripple effects on women and their families? These effects might include responses to the harm of treatment (e.g., pain, burned cervix), fears about partner reactions, fertility concerns, discomfort, and the impact of recommendations to practice abstinence for four weeks following treatment. See http://www.alliance-cxca.org/files/ACCP_FIGO_2006_Bradley.ppt#282,17; accessed April 2010.

56 In some studies of HPV infection in large populations, however, there is evidence of a second wave of new HPV infections among postmenopausal women, presumably due to exposure to new sexual partners. F. X. Bosch, A. Burchell, M. Schiffman, A. R. Giuliano, S. de Sanjose, L. Bruni, G. Tortolero-Luna, S. K. Kjaer, and N. Muñoz, "Epidemiology and natural history of human papillomavirus infections and type-specific implications in cervical neoplasia," *Vaccine* 2008, 26 (10): K1–K16.

57 E. Suba, "Suba responds" (letter to the editor), *American Journal of Public Health*, February 2007, 97 (2): 201–2. Examples of Pap infrastructure in developing

and middle-income countries include Costa Rica's Guanacaste project and projects in Chile and Colombia, countries that have large middle classes and are not comparable to the economic and social realities of many poor countries.

58 See http://www.cytojournal.com/article.asp?issn=1742-6413;year=2009 ;volume=6;issue=1;spage=12;epage=12;aulast=AUSTIN; accessed September 2009.

59 "Merck & Co., Inc. and QIAGEN N.V. today announced their intent to collaborate on a new program to increase access to HPV vaccination and HPV DNA testing in some of the most resource-poor areas of the world. This initiative is the first time a vaccine manufacturer and a molecular diagnostics company are collaborating to address the burden of cervical cancer with a comprehensive approach. Representing a combined value of approximately $600 million based on current U.S. prices, the commitments of Merck and QIAGEN were highlighted today among a select group of corporate initiatives announced at the annual meeting of the Clinton Global Initiative." http://www.fiercebiotech .com/press-releases/merck-and-qiagen-collaborate-accelerate-access-cervical -cancer-vaccination-and-screen; accessed September 2009.

60 The U.S. Preventive Services Task Force has called for an increase in the age at which screening is initiated and for widening the interval between screenings. http://www.uspreventiveservicestaskforce.org/uspstf/uspscerv.htm; accessed 2012.

61 Researchers recently experimented with homeless women in North America who were encouraged to collect their own vaginal smears, bypassing access problems and whatever other barriers exist to adequate primary and gynecologic care. G. Ogilvie, M. Krajden, J. Maginley, J. Isaac-Renton, G. Hislop, R. Elwood-Martin, C. Sherlock, D. Taylor, and M. Rekart, "Feasibility of self-collection of specimens for human papillomavirus testing in hard-to-reach women," *Canadian Medical Association Journal*, 2007, 177 (5): 480–83. A meta-analysis of studies of self-collected specimens revealed that their sensitivity, while inferior to clinical HPV sampling, was on par with or better than traditional cytological screening. G. S. Ogilvie, D. M. Patrick, M. Schulzer, J. W. Sellors, M. Petric, K. Chambers, R. White, J. M. FitzGerald, "Diagnostic accuracy of self-collected vaginal specimens for human papillomavirus compared to clinician collected human papillomavirus specimens: a meta-analysis," *Sexually Transmitted Infections*, 2005, 81 (3): 207–12. "Similarly, the development of a screening test that relies on women obtaining the sample themselves in the privacy of their homes could greatly enhance the acceptability of screening and concomitantly reduce the burden on clinic based services." Tsua and Pollack, "Preventing cervical cancer."

62 J. Ferguson, *Global Shadows: Africa in the Neoliberal World Order* (Durham, N.C.: Duke University Press, 2006).

63 S. Feierman, "When physicians meet: local medical knowledge and global public goods," in G. Wenzel and C. Molyneux, eds., *Evidence, Ethos and Experiment: The Anthropology and History of Medical Research in Africa* (Oxford, U.K.: Berghahn Books, 2011), 171–96.

Chapter 9

1 Compiled by PRIME Institute, University of Minnesota, for Families USA from data published by the Pennsylvania Pharmaceutical Assistance Contract for the Elderly (PACE) and data found in the Price-Chek PC published by Medi-Span

(Facts and Comparisons, Indianapolis), May 2002. I say forty-six, rather than the listed fifty, because in this top fifty were different dosages of the same drug (Families USA Foundation 2002).

2   S. M. Alibhai and P. A. Rochon, "The controversy surrounding cholesterol treatment in older people," *Geriatric Nephrology and Urology*, 1998 8 (1): 11–14; W. S. Aronow, "Should hypercholesterolemia in older persons be treated to reduce cardiovascular events?" *Journals of Gerontology Series A: Biological Sciences and Medical Sciences*, 2002, 57 (7): M411–M413; J. M. Eisenberg, "Should the elderly be screened for hypercholesterolemia?" *Archives of Internal Medicine*, 1991, 151 (6): 1063–65; J. Froom, "Blood cholesterol lowering in elderly patients," *Journal of the American Board of Family Practice*, 1991, 4 (1): 61–62; J. C. LaRosa, "Justifying lipid-lowering therapy in persons ≥65 years of age," *American Journal of Cardiology*, 2002, 90 (12): 1330–32; M. F. Oliver, "Should we treat hypercholesterolemia in patients over 65?" *Heart*, 1997, 77 (6): 491–92; N. K. Wenger, "Usefulness of lipid-lowering therapy in elderly patients," *American Journal of Cardiology*, 2002, 90 (8): 870–71.

3   A. Gawande, "The cancer-cluster myth," *New Yorker*, February 8, 1999, 34–37.

4   New Jersey Department of Health, *Case Control Study of Childhood Cancers in Dover Township (Ocean County), NJ Vol. 1, Summary of the Final Technical Report*, 2003, http://www.state.nj.us/health/eoh/hhazweb/case-control_pdf/Volume _I/vol_i.pdf, accessed September 15, 2004.

5   Jasanoff has argued that the Environmental Protection Agency in the 1970s epitomized a new kind of public science. A central development was the EPA's shift from an emphasis on testable knowledge claims to a preoccupation with the process of knowledge production and evaluation. The credibility of an important policy-making body derived more from the open and balanced ways that its policies were produced rather than confidence in the evidentiary basis of those policies. S. Jasanoff, "Science, politics, and the recognition of expertise at EPA," *Osiris*, 1992, 7: 192–217.

6   "Blood tests for cancer," *Science News Letter*, September 13, 1947, 163.

7   H. Evanoff, N. Checkowat, N. Weiss, and L. Rosenstock, " Periodic chest X-ray for lung cancer screening: do we really know it's useless?.," abstract and presentation at the 1993 Annual Meeting of the Robert Wood Johnson Foundation Clinical Scholars Meetings, Ft. Lauderdale.

8   A. Young, *The Harmony of Illusions: Inventing Post-traumatic Stress Disorder* (Princeton: Princeton University Press, 1995).

9   J. L. Cleeman and C. Lenfant, "New guidelines for the treatment of high blood cholesterol in adults from the national cholesterol education program: from controversy to consensus," *Arteriosclerosis*, 1987, 7 (6): 649–50.

10   E. M. Armstrong, "Diagnosing moral disorder: why fetal alcohol syndrome appeared in 1973," *Social Science and Medicine*, 1998, 47 (12): 2025–42.

11   R. Aronowitz, "From myalgic encephalitis to yuppie flu: a history of chronic fatigue syndromes," in C. Rosenberg and J. Golden, eds., *Framing Disease* (New Brunswick, N.J.: Rutgers University Press, 1992), 155–84.

12   K. Wailoo, *Drawing Blood: Technology and Disease Identity in Twentieth-Century America* (Baltimore: Johns Hopkins University Press, 1997); T. Quill, M. Lipkin, and P. Greenland, "The medicalization of normal variants: the case of mitral valve prolapse," *Journal of General Internal Medicine*, 1998, 3 (3): 267–76. What has been controversial is not the existence of prolapsed valve itself or its association with later clinical problems such as valve infection, but the attribution of different cardiac and especially "constitutional" symptoms to the prolapsed valve.

13 E. L. Wynder, "Tobacco as a cause of lung cancer: some reflections," *American Journal of Epidemiology*, 1997, 146: 687–94.

14 There is a growing literature and debate about the role of lay advocacy in a wide range of health policies. Steven Epstein's analysis of AIDS activists emphasized the changing, innovative, and, in his view, generally constructive engagement between them and clinicians, investigators, and policy makers in the context of drug development, clinical research, and policy making. S. Epstein, *Impure Science: AIDS, Activism, and the Politics of Knowledge* (Berkeley: University of California Press, 1996). In contrast, Marcia Angell's analysis of the role of lay activists in the visibility of the idea that silicone breast implants cause connective tissue disease stressed the problematic alliance between these groups and personal injury lawyers, their antagonism to mainstream medical researchers and publications, and their undue power to influence federal regulators. M. Angell, *Science on Trial: The Clash of Medical Evidence and the Law in the Breast Implant Case* (New York: W. W. Norton, 1997).

15 At least ten prospective trials evaluating radiograph screening and/or sputum cytology were begun in the 1951–75 period. The studies had heterogeneous designs and goals. While some but not all studies reported significant advantages among those screened in terms of "half-way" endpoints such as greater numbers of cancers found, earlier cancer stage at diagnosis, and duration of survival from time of diagnosis, there was no consistent and clear evidence of decreased lung cancer mortality. However, the methodological weaknesses in these studies were comparable to problems in screening research in other diseases in which demand for prevention interventions continued to run high. In these other situations, e.g., mammography for women younger than fifty, weak or negative research findings in studies with methodological problems did not lead to closure of debate and falling off of medical and lay interest. In lung cancer screening, there were only a few isolated voices in the period in which screening mammography was widely diffused who argued against the conventional wisdom that screening confers no mortality benefit. See the challenge to the prior consensus posed in two later articles: G. M. Strauss, "Screening for lung cancer: an evidence-based synthesis," *Surgical Oncology Clinics of North America*, 1999, 8 (4): 747–74, and G. M. Strauss, "Randomized population trials and screening for lung cancer: breaking the cure barrier," *Cancer*, 2000, supplement 11, 89: 2399–2421). Starting in the late 1990s, there was renewed interest in lung cancer screening using new technology (e.g., spiral CAT scans) but there continued to be much less public or medical interest in this research than in breast cancer screening.

16 R. Aronowitz, "The social construction of coronary heart disease risk factors," in *Making Sense of Illness: Science, Society, and Disease* (Cambridge, U.K.: Cambridge University Press, 1998), 111–44.

17 This selective and schematic review of HRT use is based on my own clinical experiences as well as a sampling of the clinical, policy, and social science literature in this highly contentious area. I want to anticipate any objections to imagining the HRT story as anything but a biomedical success tale, because a randomized clinical trial (RCT) of this practice was done, had conclusive results, and led to practice and policy change. First, the initial results of this RCT came after two decades in which millions of women took these hormones to reduce their risk of chronic disease. In retrospect at least, there may have been room for more effective and timely types of societal scrutiny. Second, despite the remarkable success of the Women's Health Initiative (WHI) in resolving many aspects of the HRT controversy, we cannot rely on RCTs to

settle every prevention controversy in a timely manner. In addition to the long time lag necessary to detect any effects, there are also significant methodological, economic, interpretive, and ethical problems associated with RCTs that make them impossible to deploy in the study of many other preventive practices; e.g., how could one test the effectiveness of PAP smear by an RCT with a "no testing" arm given medical and popular beliefs about the test's effectiveness as a screening tool?

18 F. Albright, P. H. Smith, and A. M. Richardson, "Postmenopausal osteoporosis," *Journal of the American Medical Association*, 1941, 116: 2465–74; E. Davis, N. M. Strandjord, and L. H. Lanzl, "Estrogens and the aging process," *Journal of the American Medical Association*, 1996, 196 (3): 129–34; G. S. Gordon, "Osteoporosis diagnosis and treatment," *Texas State Journal of Medicine*, 1961, 740–47; E. Meema and S. Meema, "Prevention of postmenopausal osteoporosis by hormone treatment of the menopause," *Canadian Medical Association Journal* 1968, 99 (6): 248–51; L. E. Nachtigall, R. H. Nachtigall, R. D. Nachtigall, and R. M. Beckman, "Estrogen replacement therapy 1: a 10-year prospective study in the relationship to osteoporosis," *Obstetrics and Gynecology* 1979, 53 (3): 277–81; Alibhai and Rochon, "The controversy surrounding cholesterol treatment in older people," 11.

19 J. E. Rossouw, G. L. Anderson, R. L. Prentice, A. Z. LaCroix, C. Kooperberg, M. L. Stefanick, R. D. Jackson, S. A. Beresford, B. V. Howard, K. C. Johnson, J. M. Kotchen, and J. Ockene, "Writing group for the Women's Health Initiative Investigators. Risks and benefits of estrogen plus progestin in healthy postmenopausal women: principal results. From the Women's Health Initiative Randomized Controlled Trial," *Journal of the American Medical Association* 2002, 288 (3): 321–33.

20 E. S. Watkins, "Dispensing with aging: changing rationales for long-term hormone replacement therapy, 1960–2000," *Pharmacy in History* 2001, 43 (1): 23–37.

21 K. I. MacPherson, "The false promises of hormone replacement therapy and current dilemma," in J. Callahan, ed., *Menopause: A Midlife Passage* (Bloomington: Indiana University Press, 1993), 145–59.

22 N. Worcester and M. H. Whatley, "The selling of HRT: playing on the fear factor," *Feminist Review*, 1992, 41: 1–26.

23 Worcester and Whatley, "The selling of HRT."

24 For examples of such pharmaceutical sponsorship of research and researchers, see D. de Aloysio, M. Gambacciani, M. Meschia, F. Pansini, A. B. Modena, P. F. Bolis, M. Massobrio, G. Aiocchi, and E. Perizzi, "The effect of menopause on blood lipid and lipoprotein levels. The Icarus Study Group," *Atherosclerosis* 1999, 147 (1): 147–53; J. H. Pickar, R. A. Wild, B. Walsh, E. Hirvonen, and R. A. Lobo, "Effects of different hormone replacement regimens on postmenopausal women with abnormal lipid levels. Menopause Study Group," *Climacteric* 1998, 1 (1): 26–32; Rossouw et al., "Writing group for the Women's Health Initiative Investigators"; C. L. Varas-Lorenzo, A. Garcia-Rodriguez, C. Cattaruzzi, M. B. Troncon, L. Agostinis, and S. Perez-Gutthann, "Hormone replacement therapy and the risk of hospitalization for venous thromboembolism: a population-based study in southern Europe," *American Journal of Epidemiology*, 1998, 147 (4): 387–90; C. Varas-Lorenzo, L. A. Garcia-Rodriguez, S. Perez-Gutthann, and A. Duque-Oliart, "Hormone replacement therapy and incidence of acute myocardial infarction: a population-based nested case-control study," *Circulation*, 2000, 101 (22): 2572–78. It is difficult to gauge the extent of this influence, in part because full disclosure of possible financial conflict of interest has been

a requirement of journal editors only in recent years. For a good discussion of these issues in the context of HRT use, see I. Palmlund, "The marketing of estrogens for menopausal and postmenopausal women," *Journal of Psychosomatic Obstetrics and Gynecology*, 1997, 18 (2): 158–64.

25 R. Klein and L. J. Dumble, "Disempowering midlife women: the science and politics of hormone replacement therapy," *Women's Studies International Forum*, 1994, 17 (4): 327–44.

26 K. Hunt, "A cure for all ills? Constructions of the menopause and the chequered fortunes of hormone replacement therapy," in S. Wilkinson and C. Kitzinger, eds., *Women and Health: Feminist Perspectives* (London: Taylor and Francis, 1994), 141–65; Worcester and Whatley, "The selling of HRT."

27 American College of Physicians, "Guidelines for counseling postmenopausal women about preventive hormone therapy," *Annals of Internal Medicine* 1992, 117 (12): 1038–41; AGS Clinical Practice Committee, "Counseling postmenopausal women about preventive hormone therapy," *Journal of the American Geriatrics Society* 1996, 44: 1120–22; H. Nawaz and D. L. Katz, "American College of Preventive Medicine Practice Policy Statement. Perimenopausal and postmenopausal hormone replacement therapy," *American Journal of Preventive Medicine*, 1999, 17 (3): 250–54. Given realities such as the complexity of the data on HRT and the physician's role in prescribing and framing information about risks and benefits, the exact meaning and contours of this autonomy were and remain unclear.

28 Nawaz and Katz, "American College of Preventive Medicine Practice Policy Statement." B. J. Oddens and M. J. Boulet, "Hormone replacement therapy among Danish women aged 45–65 years: prevalence, determinants, and compliance," *Obstetrics and Gynecology* 1997, 90 (2): 269–77.

29 Rossouw et al., "Writing group for the Women's Health Initiative Investigators." The trial was stopped as a result of a complex scientific and ethical judgment about the strength and meaning of the data at a particular point in time. Although the data were by no means unambiguous, the premature ending of the trial made it very difficult, for example, to see and therefore weigh the expected benefit in preventing osteoporosis. The study seems to have been the death knell for the preventive use of these drugs and perhaps even for the wide-scale use of these drugs for the treatment of menopausal symptoms.

30 In addition to promising to ameliorate specific symptoms and risks, HRT was also marketed as way of setting the body back to normality. This is clear from the name *hormone replacement therapy*, which suggested that these drugs supplied the hormones which women had "lost." We need to be very careful about the emotional and pre-logical appeal of returning the body to some hypothesized normal and natural state via unnatural interventions, especially when supported by such semantic sleight of hand. Eventually, even the official organs of scientific research recognized these problems; in October 2002, the NIH renamed HRT as "menopausal hormone therapy." See G. Kolata, "Replacing replacement therapy," *New York Times*, October 27, 2002, WK2.

31 Regulation of privately financed research raises many complex legal and ethical issues, but it is worth noting examples in which shifting medical and popular opinion has rapidly changed the way privately financed research is carried out. I am thinking of the successful start to requiring pharmaceutical firms to make public and register in a central database the results of all clinical studies, including ones with negative results.

32 It is not clear who has the credibility and authority to make such judgments—especially given uncertain evidence and the fact that different groups stand to win or lose as a result of particular policies. However, the situation is no dif-

ferent from our current disease prevention landscape, which is to say we are in need of more transparency and greater representation of different interests in prevention policy formulation.

Chapter 10

1 E.g., the Sleep Foundation estimates that there are eighteen million people with the problem in the U.S. today. See http://sleepfoundation.org/sleep -disorders-problems/obstructive-sleep-apnea-and-sleep, accessed June 2014.

2 See the 2011 review of the state of knowledge by the U.S. Agency for Health Care Research and Quality, http://effectivehealthcare.ahrq.gov/index.cfm /search-for-guides-reviews-and-reports/?productid=685&pageaction=display product#3340, accessed June 2014.

3 For a clear discussion of these issues, see H. G. Welch, L. Schwartz, and S. Woloshin, *Overdiagnosed: Making People Sick in the Pursuit of Health* (Boston: Beacon Press, 2011).

4 See http://www.fiercebiotech.com/story/alzheimers-pipeline-whats-next /2012-08-28, accessed June 2014; Z. Corbyn, "New set of Alzheimer's trials focus on prevention," *Lancet*, 2013, 381 (9867): 614–15.

5 Another policy response for preventing and ameliorating the suffering from diseases like AD is to propose upstream population-level interventions. Targeting the social, economic, political, and environmental determinants of disease and health can have large-scale and enduring health impacts. Margaret Lock, who has written one of the most detailed and incisive critiques of current AD practices, has argued for "a largely neglected public health approach to AD prevention, one that would entail a reduction in inequalities and toxic environments, better social support, improved education, and so on, all associated with increased risk for AD. Such an approach is the only realistic way in which AD prevention can be implemented globally." See Margaret Lock's letter (*New York Review of Books*, July 10, 2014) in response to Jerome Groopman, "How memory speaks," *New York Review of Books*, May 22, 2014; Lock's letter is accessible at http://www.nybooks.com/articles/archives/2014/jul/10/what-causes -alzheimers-an-exchange/?insrc=hpma, accessed June 2014. While these policies are likely to provide positive benefits for communities and individuals, I fear that we are as ignorant about population origins of AD as we are of its pathophysiological mechanisms. Progressive public health or population health advocates can lose credibility as well as their critical edge if their proposals are not based on solid population-level science.

6 I. Hacking, "The looping effects of human kinds"; I. D. Sperber, D. Premack, and A. J. Premack, eds., *Causal Cognition: A Multi-disciplinary Approach* (Oxford: Clarendon Press, 1995), 351–82.

7 https://www.youtube.com/watch?v=AP-H3JxVyyE; accessed July 2014.

8 Surveillance, Epidemiology, and End Results Program, 1975–2005, Division of Cancer Control and Population Sciences, National Cancer Institute, 2008. See http://seer.cancer.gov/statfacts/html/prost.html, accessed June 2014.

9 Age-adjusted prostate cancer mortality rates increased after the rapid diffusion of PSA screening and later decreased to roughly historical averages. US Mortality Data 1960–2005, US Mortality Volumes 1930–1959, National Center for Health Statistics, Centers for Disease Control and Prevention, 2008. See http:// seer.cancer.gov/statfacts/html/prost.html, accessed June 2014.

10 These issues and the studies and behaviors mentioned are all discussed in my "From Skid Row to Main Street: the Bowery series and the transformation of

prostate cancer, 1951–1966," *Bulletin of the History of Medicine*, 2014, 88 (2): 287–317.

11 The doctor is featured in a film-in-progress by Johns Hopkins University linguist Bernadette Wegenstein, whose working title was "The Good Breast" when I saw excerpts at a conference entitled "The Body Plastics" at Johns Hopkins University on November 8, 2013.

12 U. Beck, W. Bonss, and C. Lau, "The theory of reflexive modernization: problematic, hypotheses and research programme," *Theory, Culture & Society*, 2003, 20 (2): 1–33, 2. Lorraine Daston ("The domestication of risk: mathematical probability and insurance, 1650–1830," in L. Kruger, L. Daston, and M. Heidelberger, eds., *The Probabilistic Revolution* [Cambridge, MA: MIT Press, 1990], 237–60), Ian Hacking (*The Taming of Chance* [Cambridge: Cambridge University Press, 1990]), and other historians and philosophers of science have provided an intellectual history of some important developments in enlightenment and postenlightenment risk-related ideas and practices that put some contemporary sociological theorizing in historical context. They show how mathematical probability became acceptable in cultural and economic life as well as in the emerging social and physical sciences. One of the most important insights is the slow erosion of determinist assumptions about social and natural regularities in the nineteenth century. Hacking argued that the "emergence of probability" and the "taming of chance" were not simply consequences of modernity but in some sense a prerequisite. Modern life, from this perspective, is the possibility of life secure from disruptions of chance. Many aspects and consequences of the nineteenth-century emergence of probability and the centrality of statistical techniques have set the stage for many dilemmas posed by contemporary health risks. The idea of "human nature" was displaced by notions of the "normal" person with dispersions from the mean. Probabilistic ideas and practices gave the state and other institutions new means to measure and control individuals.

13 Of course, there may be unintended *positive* effects. I sometimes wonder whether important positive secular trends in disease mortality are not unintended "side effects" of other risk/disease interventions or health-motivated consumption. For example, is the dramatic decline in gastric cancer mortality an unintended side effect of post–World War II antibiotic use and consumer products such as antacids and bismuth preparations, via their impact on *H. pylori* prevalence or other mechanisms? Can some of the unexplained variance in declining cardiovascular rates have similar nonspecific and unintentional explanations?

14 At the level of biological mechanism, many risk-reducing interventions might very well work by treating/curing invisible or difficult-to-visualize active disease processes rather than by forestalling their development. Some women after a breast cancer diagnosis and surgical treatment might have some small degree of residual cancer that is cured or controlled by an antiestrogen rather than being prevented from ever developing. Either way, the patient's experience is similar. The prevention/treatment boundary is inherently fuzzy and contingent on knowledge we do not necessarily have and the perspective of the person observing the situation. Similarly, in malaria, antibiotic prophylaxis, despite the name, might very well work by having enough circulating medicine to treat small numbers of cells infected by the malaria parasite rather than by destroying parasites prior to cell infection, while drug and parasite circulate in the bloodstream.

15 See S. Epstein, *Impure Science: AIDS, Activism, and the Politics of Knowledge* (Berkeley: University of California Press, 1996). Of course, hope was held out

that regulators could divine some meaning from the natural experiment of using such drugs to guide the care of people in the future.

16 http://www.ispot.tv/ad/7Ynl/enbrel-enough; accessed August 2014.

17 D. A. Asch and J. C. Hershey, "Why some health policies don't make sense at the bedside," *Annals of Internal Medicine*, 122 (1995): 846–50.

18 An article touching on the relationship between manufacturers' production and marketing practices of new vaccines and their societal costs appeared on the day I initially drafted my views on risk and trust (E. Rosenthal, "Price of prevention: vaccine prices are soaring," *New York Times*, July 3, 2014, A1). The article focused on the high costs of new and reformulated vaccines and the resulting negative impact on clinicians and patients, such as making them unaffordable to patients and loss centers for doctors. Central to rising costs has been the way mandates for school entry have led to high profits for vaccine manufacturers, the kind of "rent" situation I described in the chapter's introduction. The article pointed out that prices for some vaccines rose after inclusion in the list of mandated vaccines for school entry. One pediatrician is quoted, "We have to give it to every kid, so it's a golden ticket." Other anticompetitive aspects of vaccine marketing include arrangements where physicians agree to a gag rule, prohibiting them from disclosing how much they paid for vaccines.

19 Biomedical acceptance of expert recommendations as objective and free of conflict of interest emerges, as I argued in chapter 3 in the section on the persuasive power of randomized clinical trials, partly from a kind of "celebrity endorsement" by individuals and groups who have earned trust by acting in accordance with well-accepted scripts and upholding norms of evidence production and interpretation. This is not to say that individual consumers and clinicians cannot or do not independently examine evidence. But at some point there is a leap of faith, based on trust (actively maintained by rituals and practices), if only because there are necessarily so many things unsaid or unsubstantiated or undocumented even in the most complete scientific report.

20 The enduring controversies over chronic Lyme disease, which as I argued shaped the vaccine controversy, are fundamentally about trust in biomedical authority. I have also pointed out that despite the high levels of mistrust and incommensurate views of the disease, both expert biomedical and heterodox alternative positions share fealty to reductive models of disease. Some small step towards restoring trust might occur by acknowledging the many chinks in the biomedical models of Lyme disease pathogenesis and the human need for compassion and legitimation of suffering not explainable by current biomedical knowledge. R. Aronowitz, "Lyme disease: the social construction of a new disease and its social consequences," *Milbank Quarterly*, 1991, 69: 79–112.

21 A. Heller, *The Immortal Comedy: The Comic Phenomenon in Art, Literature, and Life* (Lanham, MD: Lexington Books, 2005), 142.

22 I am borrowing and using in a different context for different purposes the term *precautionary principle* from environmental activists who argue that the onus is on the producers of new, potentially harmful products, practices, and policies to prove their safety before disseminating them, rather than the burden of proof falling on activists to show their dangers. See, for example, Sarah Steingraber, *Living Downstream: An Ecologist Looks at Cancer and the Environment* (Reading, MA: Addison-Wesley Publishing, 1997).

23 Aronowitz, "From Skid Row to Main Street."

24 P. Orenstein, "Our feel-good war against breast cancer," *New York Times*, magazine section, April 28, 2013, 36.

25 R. Aronowitz, "The social and economic influences on medication use and

misuse," *Journal of General Internal Medicine*, 2012, 27 (12): 1580–81. Although this was a very effective maneuver, there is often an unintended cost to even the most positive risk intervention. Reducing a risk at one point often leads to new risks somewhere else. Acetaminophen is now a leading cause of adverse drug reactions, in part because it is used in so many mass-marketed over-the-counter remedies, creating the conditions for unrecognized overuse and toxicity. Acetaminophen's wide availability and low therapeutic index (i.e., toxic levels are close to therapeutic ones) also make it a common way to attempt suicide.

26 R. Aronowitz, *Making Sense of Illness: Science, Society, and Disease* (Cambridge, U.K.: Cambridge University Press, 1998).

27 A central tenet of the U.S. Affordable Care Act is mandating preventive services that would not be subject to the deductibles and high copays frequently associated with clinical services targeted at symptoms and preexisting disease. Gilbert Welch, a physician researcher and prominent critic of overdiagnosis and overtreatment, recounted the experience of one patient whose colonoscopy, because it was triggered by a positive finding on another screening test (sampling stool samples for occult blood), was considered diagnostic and not preventative and therefore subject to a costly copay and deductible. Welch pointed out the absurdity of a system that has financial disincentives for a potentially life-saving procedure, while reimbursing the same procedure in full under conditions of much less benefit, i.e., screening for disease among the healthy. G. Welch, "The problem with free health care," *New York Times*, May 1, 2014, A25.

28 These points are further elaborated in my *Unnatural History: Breast Cancer and American Society* (Cambridge: Cambridge University Press, 2007), chapter 11.

29 The scientific efficacy of many of the core examples of prevention practices in this book, e.g., PSA screening and screening mammography for women under fifty, is disputed, so I do not pay much heed to published attempts to estimate these practices' cost-effectiveness (i.e., if there is no effectiveness, one cannot estimate cost-effectiveness). The much less studied efficacy of anticipatory practices in people already diagnosed with cancer, heart disease, etc. (if only because these practices do not—yet—form a well-recognized category of therapeutics) make it even harder to find good estimates of cost-effectiveness. At one end of the spectrum, certain secondary prevention practices are probably cost-*saving*, e.g., the use of aspirin to prevent recurrence of myocardial infarction or stroke. At the other end, the very low absolute risk of tetanus makes for a very unfavorable estimate of the cost-effectiveness of mass tetanus vaccination (costing over $450,000 to yield one quality-adjusted year of life), even though there is no doubt about the scientific efficacy of vaccination. M. V. Maciosek, A. B. Coffield, J. M. McGinnis, J. R. Harris, M. B. Caldwell, S. M. Teutsch, D. Atkins, J. H. Richland, and A. Haddix, "Priorities among effective clinical preventive services: results of a systematic review and analysis," *American Journal of Preventive Medicine* 2006, 31 (1): 55–56.

30 In McKeown's formulation, "To assist us to come safely into the world and comfortably out of it, and during life to protect the well and care for the sick and disabled." T. McKeown, *The Role of Medicine: Dream, Mirage or Nemesis* (London: Nuffield Provincial Hospitals Trust, 1976), 173.

31 McKeown, *The Role of Medicine*, 140.

Index